Well-Mannered Medicine

Well-Mannered Medicine

Medical Ethics and Etiquette in Classical Ayurveda

DAGMAR WUJASTYK

OXFORD
UNIVERSITY PRESS

OXFORD
UNIVERSITY PRESS

Oxford University Press is a department of the University of Oxford.
It furthers the University's objective of excellence in research, scholarship,
and education by publishing worldwide.

Oxford New York
Auckland Cape Town Dar es Salaam Hong Kong Karachi
Kuala Lumpur Madrid Melbourne Mexico City Nairobi
New Delhi Shanghai Taipei Toronto

With offices in
Argentina Austria Brazil Chile Czech Republic France Greece
Guatemala Hungary Italy Japan Poland Portugal Singapore
South Korea Switzerland Thailand Turkey Ukraine Vietnam

Oxford is a registered trademark of Oxford University Press
in the UK and certain other countries.

Published in the United States of America by
Oxford University Press
198 Madison Avenue, New York, NY 10016

Library of Congress Cataloging-in-Publication Data
Wujastyk, Dagmar.
Well-mannered medicine : medical ethics and etiquette in classical
Ayurveda / Dagmar Wujastyk.
p. cm.
Includes bibliographical references (p.).
ISBN 978–0–19–985626–8 (hardcover) — ISBN
978–0–19–985996–2 (pbk.) — ISBN 978–0–19–985627–5 (ebook)
1. Medicine, Ayurvedic. 2. Medical ethics—India. I. Title.
R605.W85 2012
174.2′95538—dc23 2011041072

ISBN 978–0–19–985626–8
ISBN 978–0–19–985996–2

Contents

Acknowledgments

WRITING A BOOK can be a challenging undertaking, and I am grateful for the encouragement and support I have received from family, friends, and colleagues over the years. My special thanks go to Professor Konrad Klaus for his supervision of my doctoral thesis. I would also like to thank Dr. Elizabeth de Michelis, Dr. Mark Singleton, Rajashree Dhanaraj, Professor Frederick Smith, Dr. Suzanne Newcombe, Dr. Rick Weiss, Professor Martha Selby, Professor Jan Gerrit Meulenbeld, Professor Kenneth Zysk, Dr. Philipp Maas, Professor Karin Preisendanz, Katrin Wellmann, and Dr. Dominik Wujastyk, who all have contributed either directly or indirectly to this volume.

Abbreviations

Ah.	*Aṣṭāṅgahṛdayasaṃhitā*
As.	*Aṣṭāṅgasaṃgraha*
Bhel.	*Bhelasaṃhitā*
Bhāv.	*Bhāvaprakāśa*
Ca.	*Carakasaṃhitā*
Cik.	Cikitsāsthāna, or Cikitsasthāna in the case of the *Kāśyapasaṃhitā*
Hā.	*Hārītasaṃhitā*
HIML.	History of Indian Medical Literature
Ind.	Indriyasthāna
K.A.	*Kauṭilīya Arthaśāstra*
Kāś.	*Kāśyapasaṃhitā*
Madh.	Madhyakhaṇḍa
Mādh.	*Mādhavanidāna*
Manu.	*Mānavadharmaśāstra/ Manusmṛti*
MW.	Monier-Williams: A Sanskrit–English Dictionary
Ni.	Nidānasthāna
Pūrv.	Pūrvakhaṇḍa
Śā.	Śārīrasthāna
Śār.	*Śārṅgadharasaṃhitā*
Skt.	Sanskrit
Si.	Siddhisthāna
Su.	*Suśrutasaṃhitā*
Sū.	Sūtrasthāna
Utt.	Uttarasthāna, or Uttaratantra in the case of the *Suśrutasaṃhitā*

Well-Mannered Medicine

Introduction

WHEN IS IT right for a doctor to lie to a patient? What is more important: a patient's health, or his dignity? When should a patient refuse to follow the doctor's orders? What is acceptable medical risk? Whose fault is it if a patient dies under a doctor's care? Who cares for the patient? And who pays the bill ...?

About two thousand years ago, physicians in ancient India could find answers to these questions in the then new, now classic textbooks of the traditional South Asian medical system known as Ayurveda. The ayurvedic textbooks offered many guidelines on good medical practice: They defined what made a physician a good physician, or a patient a good patient. They described the formal procedures of medical education and laid out the rules for subsequent practice. They determined the duties or obligations doctors and patients had to each other, providing a catalogue of rules of professional conduct that physicians were bound to, including guidelines on appropriate interactions with both patients and colleagues. These guidelines represent the public image of physicians, providing not only information on how physicians were meant to behave in professional situations but also how they wished to be perceived by the public.

Other guidelines are obviously addressed only to physicians. These concern very specific situations in medical care, in which a tension exists between the aim of treating patients successfully and the aim of treating them in ways patients will find acceptable from a social or a religious point of view. Both kinds of guidelines can be traced throughout the ayurvedic treatises.

The ayurvedic tradition since the nineteenth century particularly views the compendia [*saṃhitā*] ascribed to Caraka, Suśruta, and Vāgbhaṭa, as well as those ascribed to Śārṅgadhara, Mādhava, and Bhāvamiśra, as its core texts, though other treatises are also of importance both for ayurvedic history and its practice. Written in the scholarly language of Sanskrit, these texts define the precepts of Ayurveda, not merely cataloguing the causes, nature, and effects of diseases and the *materia medica* and therapies to counteract them but also offering a wider view of human life that includes psychological, social, philosophical, and spiritual perspectives.

Ayurveda is still practiced in India today, and modern practices rely on much of what the oldest medical treatises teach. However, the ayurvedic tradition is also distinguished by its continuous literary evolution over the millennia. The classical medical compendia were commented on, added to, and sometimes even refuted. A great number of new original works were composed, amounting to an enormous corpus of literature that is supplemented by new publications even today. This impressive body of work reflects both continuity and change in medicine over a period of about two thousand years. The changes documented in ayurvedic literature include the development of new theories and treatment methods. The use of the *materia medica* changed due to the availability of plants and of other resources, and new environments and ways of living—especially urbanization—changed the basic assumptions of the older texts. However, certain themes recur in many ayurvedic works, and these represent continuity within a changing tradition.[1]

In this study, I explore whether the moral and conventional discourses about the practice of medicine as described in the Sanskrit medical classics are one of these strands of continuity in ayurvedic thought. My initial question is whether there exists a medical ethic that is specific to Ayurveda, that is, whether the classical ayurvedic treatises share basic ethical assumptions about good and bad medical practice that would allow us to speak of an ayurvedic medical ethic. I use the term "ethic" as a synonym for morality and understand it to mean the principles of right and wrong that are accepted by an individual or a social group and that govern appropriate conduct. An ethical or moral code is the systematic formulation of these principles. Medical ethics, in turn, describe the moral values and rules that apply specifically to the practice of medicine.

Some rules of behavior may be based on customs or conventions of behavior rather than on moral principles. These are considered etiquette rather than ethics. The term "etiquette" is often used to describe the reciprocal interactions of persons belonging to one professional group. However, here it is used in a broader sense to describe the conventional code of practice followed by members of the medical profession toward both their peers and their patients.

Because of the wide scope of the ayurvedic works, which include discourses on various areas of philosophy, including ethics, it is necessary to differentiate between ayurvedic medical ethics and ayurvedic ethics. While ayurvedic medical ethics apply specifically to ethical questions and rules in a medical setting, they may be informed by the theoretical background and ethical reasoning of a more comprehensively formulated ayurvedic ethic. The issue of whether there exists a specifically ayurvedic medical ethic therefore encompasses three sets of questions: First, whether the guidelines on good conduct in a medical setting found in the various ayurvedic sources actually cohere with each other, allowing us to speak of an ayurvedic medical ethic in the first place (rather than of, for example, the medical ethics of Caraka, or of Vāgbhaṭa). Second, whether they are part of an ethic that only applies to medical practice or part of one that applies to human conduct in general, that is, whether ayurvedic medical ethics are separated from ayurvedic ethics in the texts. Third, whether the moral discourses on good medical practice found in the ayurvedic treatises are unique to the ayurvedic tradition or whether they have parallels in other sources, or are inspired by other disciplines or traditions.

Several modern publications dealing with ethics in the ayurvedic works compare ancient Greek concepts of medical ethics with those found in the ayurvedic treatises, finding a number of similarities between them. Julius Jolly (1994 [1951], 22–23), for example, specifically noted parallels between "the characterization of the physicians and the directions given to them reminding us of the oath of the Asclepiads" (i.e., the Hippocratic Oath).[2] It makes sense to compare the ayurvedic works with Greek sources, since both similarities with Greek humoral theory, as well as with some other aspects of pathology, and the fact that there is mention of Indian plants in Greek medical literature (though none of Greek medicines in ayurvedic literature) suggest some form of exchange between Greek and South Asian medicine.[3] The exact nature of this contact, however, remains a subject of speculation, as there is no mention in either Greek or Sanskrit literature of contact or exchange with physicians from the other culture. In the case of medical ethics, I believe the similarities with Greek medicine to be superficial, since, as I hope to show, the ethical guidelines propounded in the Sanskrit medical treatises very much follow customs and beliefs that are specific to a South Asian cultural context, with links to or at least parallels with both brahmanic and Buddhist thought.

The definition suggested above of "ethics" as the principles of right and wrong that are accepted by an individual or a social group and that govern appropriate conduct means that ethics are relative: The categories of right and wrong, or good and bad may mean very different things to different persons, let alone persons from different social or cultural backgrounds, different societies, or indeed different times. In the case of ethics expressed in the ayurvedic classics, we are looking at a very long period in time, an only vaguely circumscribed but probably quite large geographical area, and a great range of political and social backgrounds. As a body of literature, the ayurvedic works span about two thousand years, the ones examined in this study about fifteen hundred years—a time frame that hardly allows for a homogenous narrative of social and political circumstances. It is not all that clear when and where and in what kinds of society the authors of the ayurvedic classics lived. There is insufficient information on the dates and places the works were written, and hardly any biographical data for the authors. The ayurvedic treatises themselves offer little in the way of concrete information on the places, times, and contexts in which they were written. In any case, each of the earlier works underwent a series of revisions over several centuries, so that one can hardly point to one particular time and place (and hence political or social structure) for even one single work.

Taking all this into consideration, it seems ludicrous to conceive of a pan-ayurvedic ethic with a coherent set of moral principles and etiquette to begin with. On the other hand, the ayurvedic compendia are part of a tradition that takes its cues from its past, and this lets the ayurvedic treatises speak more or less in one voice on many of their subjects. The authors of the *Carakasaṃhitā* and the *Suśrutasaṃhitā* compiled their treatises from similar materials. Vāgbhaṭa expressly stated that his *Aṣṭāṅgahṛdayasaṃhitā* was a synthetical summary of the two earlier works. The later works quote copiously from the earlier ones, or paraphrase them: they look back to what was before. There is certainly innovation in the classical ayurvedic works, and they do record differences of opinion, but the fact remains that there is also a great deal of repetition and copying. This means that we can, in fact, expect certain things to stay exactly as they were when first formulated in the oldest treatises, or to be very similar. Indeed, this allows the ayurvedic tradition to be conceived as a tradition in the first place.

However, one might expect the ethics of medical practice to be rather more subject to change than other aspects of medicine. By definition, ethics should reflect the moral assumptions of the societies that formulate them. Since physicians could hardly have become an independent society unto themselves due to the interactive nature of their work, it seems reasonable to expect that the norms for medical practice were adapted to the common rules of good behavior and the moral principles of whatever communities physicians lived in.

We know that there was a great deal of change in South Asia over the period in which the ayurvedic works were written, with various competing kingdoms fighting for hegemony and social dominance, borders moving constantly, political and religious allegiances changing along with the dominant ruling powers. Bearing this in mind, we should expect to see changes in the ayurvedic authors' expressions of their medical ethics. However, my research shows that these authors hardly diverge from each other in their descriptions of good medical practice. As noted, this does not come entirely as a surprise. The sample of works that I examine in this study are, after all, closely related, which is partly the reason why they are now considered core treatises of the classical ayurvedic tradition.

And yet, could a physician in the sixteenth century in Bengal really have had the same answers to ethical questions—or indeed, even the same questions—as his predecessor in the first century in Kashmir? Or does the lack of change in this area of Ayurveda signify something else? The apparent disregard for political and social change is a phenomenon that is not specific to the ayurvedic tradition: We encounter it throughout Sanskrit literature. Sheldon Pollock (1989, 606) has succinctly described the phenomenon:

> To an astonishing degree Sanskrit texts are anonymous or pseudonymous, or might just as well be. The strategy of eliminating from the text—whatever sort of text it might be—the personality of the author and anything else that could help us situate the text in time is a formal correlate of a content invariably marked by ahistoricality. Works on statecraft, for example, describe their subject without specific reference to a single historically existing state. Books on law expatiate on such crucial questions as the relationship between local practices and general codes of conduct without adducing any particularized events or cases. Belles-lettres seem virtually without date or place, or indeed, author. Literary criticism prior to the tenth century (Ānandavardhana) neither mentions the name nor cites the work of any poet, the alaṃkārikas themselves supplying all examples. Philosophical disputation takes place without the oppositional interlocutor ever being named and doxographies make no attempt to ascribe the religious-philosophical doctrines they review to anyone, unless a mythological personage.... In short, we can read thousands of pages of Sanskrit on any imaginable subject and not encounter a single passing reference to a historical person, place, or event—or at least to any that, historically speaking, matters.

The classical ayurvedic works are part of a genre of Sanskrit literature called *śāstra*, that is, works about technical or specialized knowledge. These works represent a certain type of learning that links itself with the Vedas, the ancient brahmanic liturgical scriptures. This link is established in a number of ways, often through the simple device of directly stating a connection with Vedic knowledge, by referring to common content, or by positing a lineage of knowledge transfer that goes back to the Vedas or to divinities or sages associated with them. Pollock (1989, 609–610) states that there is, in fact, hardly any branch of Sanskritic learning whose texts do not claim authority by asserting a quasi-Vedic status in one way or another. This is the context for Pollock's explanation of why so much of Sanskrit literature typically lacks historical references. His argument is based on the Veda exegesis of the Mīmāṃsa school of thought. Mīmāṃsa is one of the six orthodox Hindu philosophies and is concerned with the nature of *dharma* (here in the sense of objective truth) based on close hermeneutics of the Vedas. According to Mīmāṃsa philosophy, the nature of *dharma* isn't accessible to reason or observation, and must be inferred from the authority of the revelation contained in the Vedas, which are considered eternal, authorless, and infallible. Pollock suggests that the Mīmāṃsakas' propositions regarding the nature of the Veda and its relation to accessing *dharma* are at the root of the ahistoricality of brahmanic intellectual discourses. One of the axiomatic claims of the Mīmāṃsakas is that the transcendence of the Vedas is confirmed by the lack of historical references within them. This leads to a somewhat circular argument: *Dharma* is transcendent and can only be accessed through transcendent forms of knowledge. The Veda is transcendent, therefore it has no author and no beginning and no reference to things that occur in time and in place. Therefore, anonymity and a lack of reference to specific times and places are markers of transcendence, and thus indicative of a text (or a body of knowledge) being a means to understanding *dharma*.

The validity of knowledge therefore partly rests on its not being placed in a specific context of time and place. According to Pollock, this notion had repercussions for the wider brahmanic intellectual enterprise, as it became a model for how to represent knowledge, or indeed what kind of knowledge was worth representing in the first place. Since "the Vedas were emptied of their 'referential intention,' other sorts of Brahmanical intellectual practices seeking to legitimate their truth-claims had perforce to conform to this special model of what counts as knowledge, and so to suppress the evidence of their own historical existence" (Pollock, 1989, 609).

In the case of the ayurvedic treatises, then, their authors would have been copying a certain format of expression that established their texts as part of orthodox brahmanic learning.[4] The conservative nature of the ethical guidelines would have confirmed the orthodox status of the texts. Correspondingly, physicians using these textbooks would have been perceived as practicing an orthodox type of medicine, perhaps even independently of whether they actually adhered to the rules or not. Therefore, while the actual ethical guidelines may not have applied to a physician's actual practice of medicine, they would still have had a vital function for medical practice in establishing the status of medicine and of physicians in society.

There is another point to consider, namely that we may be dealing with an altogether different conception of history. Deshpande (1993, xiv) argues that the ancient classical tradition believed in mythical versions of history, the core of which was that cycles of the existence of the world begin with creation and end in its destruction and that within these cycles, there is "an inevitable progression from an initial golden age of purity and truth to the final age of universal strife, which ends in the destruction of the world." We encounter this very idea in the *Carakasaṃhitā*, and I discuss its implications for medical ethics in chapter 6. Deshpande (xv) contended that this perspective on history meant that "in order to maintain a certain level of purity in the world, one needs to at least freeze certain stages of history and guard them against further change, if one cannot ideally reverse the direction of the inevitable degenerative transformation." Accordingly, ayurvedic medical ethics would be a frozen version of an ideal belonging to better times. This does not, however, tell us whether these ideals continued to influence actual medical practice or whether they were simply symbolic of an exalted idea of rightness. It is easy to imagine a mismatch between the ideals of theory and the reality of practice, between a pandit's *śāstric* learning and the nitty-gritty of medical encounters, but it is not automatically a given. This is an area that is open to further questioning.[5]

Literature on Medical Ethics in Ayurveda

A number of publications also deal with the aspects of Ayurveda discussed in this study. Among the most heavily researched topics that I will discuss is the medical student's initiation, which is described in the *Carakasaṃhitā* (Vimānasthāna 8), in the *Suśrutasaṃhitā* (Sūtrasthāna 2–4, with additional relevant passages in Sūtrasthāna 9.3 and 10.3–4, and 9), in the *Aṣṭāṅgasaṃgraha* (Sūtrasthāna 2.1–20), and in the Vimānasthāna of the *Kāśyapasaṃhitā*.[6] The medical student's initiation is relevant to a study on medical ethics because its description in some cases includes guidelines on the moral duties of the student and the physician. The most recent and probably most thorough publication dealing with the medical student's initiation is by Karin Preisendanz (2007). Her article gives a detailed structural analysis of the passage in Caraka's Vimānasthāna 8, together with comparisons to the passages mentioned above in the *Suśrutasaṃhitā* and the *Kāśyapasaṃhitā*, but with some reference also to the *Hārītasaṃhitā*, the *Bhelasaṃhitā*, and the *Aṣṭāṅgasaṃgraha*. Preisendanz gives a clear overview of how the passage is situated within the Vimānasthāna, within the *Carakasaṃhitā* as a whole, and within ayurvedic literature and briefly touches on its parallels with brahmanic literature. A further article on the latter topic is currently under preparation.[7] Preisendanz (2007, 634–638) provides a thorough survey of publications on the medical student's initiation, which

I summarize here, adding sources that concern the wider issue of medical ethics.

One of the earliest mentions in modern scholarly literature of the ayurvedic physician's professional conduct occurs in Whitelaw Ainslie's *Materia Medica of Hindoostan*, published in 1813. Ainslie argued that Hindu physicians had been misrepresented in previous publications, where they had been depicted as unlearned pretenders.[8] Ainslie's own experience led him to the opposite evaluation: "Not a few of them have I known, who were not only intimately acquainted with all the medical *Sastrums*, great part of which they had by heart; but who in other respects, were in their lives and manners correct, obliging and communicative."[9] In this, Ainslie concurs with Sir William Jones, whom he quotes as follows:

> All the tracts on medicine must indeed be studied by the Vydyas, (Doctors) and they have often more learning, and far less pride, than any of the Brahmins. They are usually Poets, Grammarians, Rhetoricians and Moralists; and may in fact be esteemed the most virtuous and amiable of the Hindoos.[10]

Jones's and Ainslie's (and Sonnerat's and Heyne's) views reflect Western perceptions of Indian physicians and medicine in their times. Jones and Ainslie, however, seem to have equated the Indian ayurvedic doctor of their times with the physician as described in ancient medical texts. Thus, to substantiate his and Jones's claim that Hindu physicians were learned scholars with a steady set of morals, Ainslie cited the following passage from a Tamil medical work that he called the "Aghastier Vytia Anyouroo":[11]

> *What constitutes a good physician.* The sages (*maharshies*) have thus handed down to us the qualities which constitute a good physician: he must be a person of strict veracity, and of the greatest sobriety and decorum, holding sexual intercourse with no woman, except his own wife: he ought to be thoroughly skilled in all the commentaries on the *ayurveda*, and be otherwise a man of sense and benevolence; his heart must be charitable; his temper calm; and his constant study how to do good. Such an individual is properly called a good physician, and such a physician ought still daily to improve his mind by an attentive perusal of scientific books (vaghadum).
>
> When a patient expresses himself peevishly or hastily, a Vytian, so endowed, will not thereby be provoked to impatience; he remains mild, yet courageous, and cherishes a cheerful hope of being able to save the

> sufferer's life; he is frank, communicative, impartial and liberal, yet ever rigid in exacting an adherence to whatever regimen or rules he may think it necessary to enjoin. Should death come upon us, under the care of this earthly saint, it can only be considered as inevitable fate, and not the consequence of presumptuous ignorance.

The reference to "vaghadum" would seem to indicate that either the "Aghastier Vytia Anyouroo" quotes from one of the works ascribed to Vāgbhaṭa (i.e., the *Aṣṭāṅgahṛdayasaṃhitā* or the *Aṣṭāṅgasaṃgraha*) or that this Tamil treatise is, in fact, a translation of one of, or part of, one of these works. However, I can only find slight similarities of the above-cited passages with passages of related content in the *Aṣṭāṅgasaṃgraha*.[12] It is not quite clear how Ainslie obtained the quotations above, that is, whether they were his own translations or someone else's. In any case, his brief discussion represents one of the earliest attempts in modern scholarship to grapple with the textual evidence for professional ethics in Ayurveda.

The next, even more brief mention of a topic related to ayurvedic professional ethics occurs in 1823, in Horace H. Wilson's essay "Medical and Surgical Sciences of the Hindus." In this summary of Hindu medical sciences, which is based on extracts from the *Suśrutasaṃhitā*, we find some discussion on what skills made the ancient Indian physician a good physician. Wilson noted that both a thorough grounding in medical theory as well as in medical practice were required of the ayurvedic physician of old, and gave an account of the training methods employed to gain the required skills.[13] The emphasis on knowledge and skill found in most of the Sanskrit medical treatises constitutes the foundation of the ayurvedic physician's ethics, as I discuss later.

The first more detailed study of medical ethics in the ayurvedic classics can be found in Thomas Wise's *Commentary on the Hindu System of Medicine* of 1845. Based on translations of the *Carakasaṃhitā* and the *Suśrutasaṃhitā*,[14] it includes chapters on the rank of physicians and duties of teachers; on the character and duties of pupils; on the duties of the physician, of the attendants, and of the patient; and on the recompense of the physician.[15]

Rudolph Roth's 1872 translation into German of Vimānasthāna 8 and of Sūtrasthāna 29 of the *Carakasaṃhitā* made these text passages, which are about medical study and about quacks, respectively, available to a wider readership for the first time. Roth's translation formed the basis for Theodor Puschmann's chapter "Medical Teaching in Ancient Times. India" in his 1891 volume *A History of Medical Education from the Most Remote to the Most Recent Times*. Puschmann also refers to the relevant passages in the *Suśrutasaṃhitā* as described in Thomas Wise's book.

Bhagvat Sinh Jee's *Short History of Aryan Medical Science* (1896) includes a chapter on the qualities of a physician. Based on a number of Sanskrit medical treatises (though Sinh Jee did not give references),[16] as well as on Sinh Jee's knowledge of contemporary practices, the chapter encompasses discussions of the physician's remuneration, his professional behavior, diagnosis and prognosis, and the signs of a patient's imminent death.

In 1897, Gustave Liétard published his comparative study "Le médicin Charaka. Le serment des hippocratistes et le serment des médicins hindous," which was based on Roth's study of Caraka's Vimānasthāna. Liétard had already written about medical education and practice in ancient India in 1858 in his doctoral thesis, "Essai sur l'histoire de la médicine chez les Indous," and again in 1862, in "Lettre historiques sur la médicine chez les Indous" and "Suşruta" (1864?).[17] For these, Liétard relied on Wise's *Commentary* as well as on the translation of the *Suśrutasaṃhitā* into Latin by Franz Hessler (1844–55). All three essays describe passages in the medical treatises that deal with morality in medicine, and specifically with a medical student's conduct during his apprenticeship and a physician's professional conduct once the apprenticeship is concluded. Liétard particularly emphasized the similarities between South Asian and Greek medicine, concluding that the latter influenced the former.

Palmyr Cordier, a junior colleague of Liétard, also wrote about medical education in ancient India in his essay "L'enseignement médical dans l'Inde ancienne. Temps védico-brahmaniques." Cordier used Buddhist sources, such as the Pāli Canon (particularly the *Jātakas* (stories about the rebirths of the Buddha), and the *Mahāvagga*, which is part of the Canon's Vinaya (i.e., monastic rules) section, as well as the medical treatises of Caraka, Suśruta, Vāgbhaṭa, Hārīta, and others, comparing them with Sanskrit religious law literature.[18]

Julius Jolly's 1901 monograph *Medicin* includes chapters on the training of physicians and on their position and practice. These chapters, which are based on readings from the compendia of Caraka and Suśruta, as well as on their commentaries, deal with such topics as quacks, the aim of physicians to become royal physicians, whom a physician should treat for free, and how a physician should behave in general. This book was translated into English and updated by C. G. Kashikar in 1951, when it was published under the title *Indian Medicine*, and remains in print today.

Henry Zimmer's posthumously published *Hindu Medicine*, which was based on two lectures he had given as part of a lecture series in 1940, discusses many topics relevant to medical ethics. Among these are the description of medical education and the relationship between master and pupil; the reasons for studying and practicing medicine; the initiation of the medical student;

professional conduct; and definitions of the good doctor, patient, medicine, and attendant.[19]

Radha Kumud Mookerji's 1947 *Ancient Indian Education: Brahmanical and Buddhist* includes sections on medical education, with descriptions of the rules of medical study, the student's initiation, the qualifications of a physician, and the factors of success in treatment (i.e., the four pillars of treatment: the doctor, the nurse (or attendant), the patient, and the medicine).

A. L. Basham's important book *The Wonder That Was India*, first published in 1954, contains an appendix on physiology and medicine in which he discusses the ancient Indian physician's status in society and gives a translation of Ca.Vi.8.7.[20] In his article "The Practice of Medicine in Ancient and Medieval India," published in Charles Leslie's seminal *Asian Medical Systems* (1st ed. 1976), Basham expanded on this theme and also wrote about medical education, the medical student's initiation, professional conduct, the physician's relationship to the king, and medicine as public service. Basham based his analyses on the *Carakasaṃhitā*, the *Suśrutasaṃhitā*, and the *Aṣṭāṅgahṛdayasaṃhitā* but also referred to the *Kauṭilīya Arthaśāstra*, Manu's *Dharmaśāstra*, and some Buddhist sources.

The joint work *Surgical Ethics in Āyurveda* by the physician G. D. Singhal and the ayurvedic doctor Damodar Sharma Gaur, published in 1963, is a compilation of passages from the Sanskrit medical treatises (the *Carakasaṃhitā*, the *Suśrutasaṃhitā*, the *Aṣṭāṅgasaṃgraha*, and the *Aṣṭāṅgahṛdayasaṃhitā*). The passages, which are first given in the Sanskrit original and then translated into English, are ordered topically in nine groups: (1) General Ethics, (2) Professional and Academic Ethics, (3) Pre-operative Ethics, (4) Operative Ethics, (5) Post-operative Ethics, (6) The Ethics and Importance of Experimental Surgery, (7) Quacks, (8) Ethics towards the Dying, and (9) Ethics in Emergency Surgery. As these headings (which are supplemented by many subheadings) suggest, Singhal and Gaur cover a lot of ground in cataloguing and translating relevant text passages. The clear translations are sometimes supplemented by notes, which are, however, most often not relevant to an understanding of the text. There is no discussion or analysis of the text selections.

Debiprasad Chattopadhyaya's *Science and Society in Ancient India*, which was first published in 1977, contains discussions on the use of meat, and specifically beef, in the ayurvedic works. Chattopadhyaya noted that recommendations to eat beef sit alongside stanzas that extol the veneration of the cow, and he interpreted this paradox as one of the examples of how an unorthodox science, that is, medicine, had received a—somewhat unconvincing—veneer of brahmanical orthodoxy. In the context of the use of meat and the physician's use of deception to make a patient eat medically beneficial but socially unacceptable substances,[21] Chattopadhyaya defined the medical ethics of a physician as follows: "What concerns him is medicine and medicine alone. If therefore there is any direct clash between medicine and morality in its abstract sense, the physician cannot help choose the former."[22]

I. A. Menon and H. F. Haberman's 1979 essay "The Medical Students' Oath of Ancient India" is among the best known and most cited articles that discuss the teacher's speech at the initiation of the medical student. It is here that the mistake of conflating the teacher's speech with a student's oath was introduced. Menon and Haberman translate and discuss Ca.Vi.8.13–14 (though only part of 14, i.e., up to the student's avowal to abide by the teacher's rules), dividing the teacher's speech into topical sections. This division has been criticized by Preisendanz (2007, 637–638).[23]

Ramachandra Rao's *Encyclopedia of Indian Medicine* (vol. 2, "Basic Concepts"), published in 1987, has a number of entries that deal with medical ethics: See, for example, "Discussions (Clinical)," "Four Props of Medical Practice" (on definitions of physicians, patients, attendants, and medicines), "Medical Ethics" (essentially a summary of Ca.Vi.8.8–13, i.e., the teacher's speech to the student on the occasion of the medical student's initiation), "The physician" (on good physicians and quacks), and "Vaidya" (reiterating the entry "The Physician").

Francis Zimmermann's book *The Jungle and the Aroma of Meats: An Ecological Theme in Hindu Medicine,* first published in 1987 and now a classic reading for anyone undertaking studies in Indian medicine, contains discussions of the themes of violence in medicine, vegetarianism, honesty, friendship, and compassion.

Julius Lipner's essay "The Classical Hindu View on Abortion and the Moral Status of the Unborn" of 1989 looks at the wider frame of Hindu literature, and it contains a concise summary of what can be found on the topic of abortion in the ayurvedic classics.

Gérard Huguet's doctoral thesis, "La Médecine Indienne Traditionelle et le Fin de la Vie: Considerations Éthiques et Medicales Intérêt Pratique Actuel," submitted in 1993 at the University of Bordeaux, discusses the discourses concerning patients' end of life in the *Carakasaṃhitā* and the *Suśrutasaṃhitā*. Among the topics explored are longevity, quality of life, incurable diseases and palliative care, and euthanasia. Huguet also summarized the contents of Ca.Vi.8.13–14 (i.e., the teacher's speech concerning the student's conduct during and after his apprenticeship). Huguet based his analysis entirely on the often imprecise English translations of the medical texts by P. V. Sharma, R. K. Sharma, B. Dash, K. Bhishagratna, and I. A. Menon and H. F. Haberman.

Prakash N. Desai's 1989 *Health and Medicine in the Hindu Tradition* includes a chapter on Ayurveda (both ancient and modern), in which he discusses topics such as the doctor–patient relationship, the status of the ayurvedic physician, ayurvedic education, the moral requirements of the medical student, caring, and curing. In another chapter, Desai explores the ayurvedic views on death and dying, and on madness. Desai also published an article on medical ethics in South and South East Asia in Warren Thomas Reich's *Encyclopedia of Bioethics*, which covers many of the same topics.[24]

Guy Mazars's short introduction to Ayurveda of 1995, *La médecine indienne*, has a chapter on the medical profession, which includes descriptions of medical education, ayurvedic ethics, and the physician's status in ancient Indian society.[25] The book was translated into English and published under the title *A Concise Introduction to Indian Medicine* in 2006.

The short monograph *Doctor–Patient Relationship in Ancient Indian Medicine (Ayurveda)* by G. S. Lavekar, published in 1996, is a compilation of text passages from mostly the *Carakasaṃhitā* and the *Suśrutasaṃhitā*, with brief discussions of their contents. Lavekar also gives the Sanskrit references for the passages he translates or paraphrases. His selection of text passages is fairly comprehensive and a useful guide to what the treatises contain on the subject matter of the doctor–patient relationship. However, the book does not offer a critical analysis of the chosen extracts and is also written in somewhat faulty, though comprehensible, English.

Bhagwan Dash's *Fundamentals of Ayurvedic Medicine* contains a chapter on study and practice, which paraphrases the beginning of Vimānasthāna 8 of the *Carakasaṃhitā*, and therefore includes the topics of how to choose a textbook, how to choose a suitable student and teacher, and the student's initiation. There is also a description of the three kinds of physician (real, feigned, and fraudulent, according to Ca.Sū.11.50–53), of the attributes of a good physician (see Ca.Sū.29.3–8) and of quacks (see Ca.Sū.29.8–9).

Dominik Wujastyk's *Roots of Ayurveda*, first published in 1998, provides translations and discussions of several passages that deal with themes of medical ethics, such as the professional conduct of physicians and of medical staff. I reproduce and discuss several of these translations in this study.

Albert A. Jonsen's *Short History of Medical Ethics* (2000) devotes a chapter to the medical ethics of India and China.[26] The part devoted to India discusses such topics as the moral purpose of medical practice, the physician's professional conduct, and the so-called Oath of Caraka (i.e., the teacher's speech in Ca.Vi.8.13–14).

Hartmut Scharfe's 2002 monograph *Education in Ancient India* also discusses medical education, and in that context explores the relationship between master and pupil and the initiation of the medical student, including the moral injunctions of the teacher's speech.

Charles Malamoud's article "Doctors as Characters in Sanskrit Literature" (2002) reflects on the ways physicians and their status are depicted in Sanskrit literature, and how these depictions tally with the self-representation of physicians in the medical classics.

M. S. Valiathan's *Legacy of Caraka* (2003), which is a summary and discussion of the contents of the *Carakasaṃhitā*, has chapters on the practice of medicine; learning to be a physician (which describes the criteria for eligibility to study, the student's initiation, and his academic preparation); a physician's calling; the medical quartet (i.e., the four pillars of treatment); genuine and fraudulent physicians; a physician's training in theory and practice; and the ethics of medical practice. Similarly, Valiathan's *Legacy of Suśruta* (2007) provides chapters on comparable topics as they arise in the *Suśrutasaṃhitā*. There is, for example, a chapter on the initiation and training of physicians that describes the moral expectations of a student and a physician.

Athavale and Athavale's short monograph *The Ideal Physician* (2003) was written to "give the guidelines as to how to become an ideal physician as per concepts of Ayurveda."[27] To this end, the authors give Sanskrit quotations from the *Suśrutasaṃhitā*, the *Carakasaṃhitā*, the *Kāśyapasaṃhitā*, and some other, nonmedical sources. However, the quotations are neither translated nor paraphrased but simply set in more or less relevant passages that discuss a number of topics, such as the definition of a useful and happy life, health, the purpose of teaching and studying Ayurveda, and so on. The usual text passages are paraphrased, such as those describing the medical student's initiation and the four pillars of treatment. The booklet is full of assertions that cannot be verified from a reading of the texts,[28] and for this reason only of limited use for a critical study of ayurvedic medical ethics, although it contains much of the relevant source material.

Cromwell Crawford, in his *Hindu Bioethics for the Twenty-First Century* (2003), sought to answer the question what a Hindu response would be to modern bioethical issues such as cloning, contraception, prenatal diagnosis, maximizing the quality of later life, death and dying, and population growth. To this end, Crawford looked to ancient Indian sources, including the ayurvedic treatises. One chapter is specifically dedicated to Ayurveda, though reference is made throughout to ayurvedic sources. In the section on Indian medicine, Crawford discussed the issues of determinism and freedom,[29] the professionalisation of the *Vaidya*, that is, the ayurvedic physician, the ayurvedic treatises' descriptions of quacks, medical education, the student's initiation,[30] and medical licensing. Crawford's interpretation of the sources is biased toward creating an image of a uniformly sympathetic and caring medical milieu. For example, in the chapter "Ayurveda on Death with Dignity," Crawford argues (in line with Prakash Desai) that the ayurvedic dictum not to treat patients who are about to die is based on moral grounds (though also bolstered by considerations of professional interest).[31] However, a close reading of the medical treatises shows that the medical authors do not provide any moral reasoning for their prohibition against treating the terminally ill, nor do they discuss the concept of a dignified death in any way (see my discussion of this topic in chapter 4).

In my own article (published in 2005 under my maiden name, Benner) "The Medical Ethics of Professionalized Ayurveda," I discussed the links (or rather, lack of links) between the ethical values expressed in the ayurvedic classics with the codified ethics of the modern ayurvedic establishment in India today. The findings of my study must be revised to some extent, since the new government-approved syllabus for students of Ayurveda in India, issued in 2009 by the Central Council for Indian Medicine, now includes modules on the ethics of classical Ayurveda. Therefore, the medical ethics of the classical tradition of Ayurveda still—or perhaps more accurately, again—play a role in the education of ayurvedic students. Since the values propounded in the ayurvedic classics form part of the modern ayurvedic syllabus, students should at least have an idea of what was important to the ancient authors. However, they are not officially required to apply these traditional ethics to their own practice. Instead, the CCIM, the regulatory body for the practice of Ayurveda in India, stipulates that practitioners of Ayurveda must follow its official guidelines to become registered doctors. These guidelines were developed by the World Medical Association (WMA). At the time the guidelines were issued, the WMA was constituted only of physicians of modern medicine, and the sources they looked to for guidance in formulating their official code of ethics were historically connected with their medicine.[32] The official medical ethics of modern Ayurveda, therefore, are based on tenets derived from a different cultural and historical background.

Finally, there are a number of short articles that discuss medical ethics in both ancient and modern India. See for example, the encyclopedia entry by O. P. Jaggi (1982), "Medical Ethics, History of: India," the article "Medical Ethics in India: Ancient and Modern," by C. M. Francis (1997), published in the online journal *Issues in Medical Ethics*, and the essay "Medical Ethics in India: Then and Now," by S. K. Pandya (1999) in the journal *Neurosurgery and Medical Ethics*.

Only few of the aforementioned works are dedicated solely or even mainly to aspects of medical ethics in Ayurveda. Most of the excerpts from the ayurvedic treatises that deal with aspects of medical ethics are presented in the context of a general summary of the tenets of Indian (i.e., South Asian) medicine. The majority of publications offer translations, paraphrases, and summaries of the relevant passages but do not necessarily discuss their contents.

The early modern scholarly publications on Indian medicine were written by medical doctors (for example, Ainslie, Heyne, Wise, Liétard, and Cordier), some of whom were interested in finding materials in ayurvedic literature that would be useful for modern medical practice. It seems that these writers felt they had to make a case for the validity of studying Indian medicine, and their attempts to put Ayurveda into context with Greek medicine may be understood as part of this endeavor. In later publications, the quest for medically useful ayurvedic knowledge seems to have been abandoned in favor of studying Indian medicine as part of the wider context of South Asian culture and history.[33] The studies by Jolly, Zimmer, Mookerji, Basham, Chattopadhyaya, Menon and Haberman, Zimmermann, Lipner, Mazars, Wujastyk, and Malamoud belong to this category. Puschmann's and Jonsen's contributions on Indian medicine place it within the context of world history. A further group of publications is based on the idea that ayurvedic thought is relevant to modern-day life, and that much can be learnt from its tenets by both practitioners of biomedicine and a lay readership. The studies by Singhal and Gaur, Athavale and Athavale, Valiathan, Lavekar, Pandya, Crawford, and Desai belong to this category, and particularly the last three are examples of the attempt to apply ancient values to modern cultural forms.

Source Texts

The Main Source Texts

As noted, a number of textbooks are regarded as foundational works of Ayurveda. A tradition exists of calling the two earliest ayurvedic works, the *Carakasaṃhitā* and the *Suśrutasaṃhitā*, together with Vāgbhaṭa's *Aṣṭāṅga-hṛdayasaṃhitā* (or, according to others, the *Aṣṭāṅgasaṃgraha*)[34] the "great threesome" (*bṛhattrayī*) of Ayurveda.

The *Carakasaṃhitā* is, at least in parts, considered to be the oldest of the classical medical treatises. It is an encyclopaedic work on medicine that is largely devoted to internal medicine (*kāyacikitsā*). Its history is complicated, and an authoritative dating of the treatise is not possible. There is reference to a physician called Caraka at the court of Kaniṣka (who is thought to have ruled the Kushan empire in the second century CE) in a late fifth-century Chinese translation of a Sanskrit text (the original of which has been lost). However, in the compendium, Caraka is only referred to as the editor of the *Agniveśatantra* (Agniveśa's treatise). In other words, not Caraka but Agniveśa is credited with writing the original text, which may be much older than Caraka's revision of it. We do not have any concrete information on Agniveśa. Caraka's revision of Agniveśa's work was reworked again by Dṛḍhabala, who probably lived in the fourth or fifth century. Dṛḍhabala seems to have contributed his own writing to the *Carakasaṃhitā*. He is named as the author at the endings of a number of chapters. The *Carakasaṃhitā* only begins to be quoted widely in other parts of Sanskrit literature in the fourth and fifth centuries.[35] According to Meulenbeld (1999–2002, IA, 114), affinity to Vaiśeṣika philosophy, but also to Nyāya, suggests that "the author called Caraka cannot have lived later than about A.D. 150–200 and not much earlier than about 100 B.C."[36]

The *Suśrutasaṃhitā* is an encyclopaedic work on medicine that covers many of the same fields as the *Carakasaṃhitā* but has a special emphasis on surgery. As for its date, the situation is similarly uncertain. There is a very early reference to the name Suśruta in a grammatical work dated around. 250 BCE, and clear reference to the *Suśrutasaṃhitā* in the Bower manuscript, which is dated to the sixth century CE.[37] Similar to the *Carakasaṃhitā*, the *Suśrutasaṃhitā* is usually regarded as a work of two or more strata that belong to different periods. The tradition that an original treatise by a historical Suśruta was later revised and transformed into the *Suśrutasaṃhitā* as we know it is already found in the commentaries of Cakrapāṇidatta (eleventh century CE) and Ḍalhaṇa (twelfth century CE). The identity of this reviser, his date, and the question whether or not the same reviser added the Uttaratantra (the last chapter of the *Suśrutasaṃhitā*) to an earlier version ending with the Kalpasthāna are controversial issues.[38] Wujastyk (2003, 64) concludes: "we have a work the kernel of which probably started some centuries BC in the form of a text mainly on surgery, but which was then heavily revised and added to in the centuries before AD 500."

The *Aṣṭāṅgahṛdayasaṃhitā* (The compendium of the heart of medicine) describes itself as a synthesis of the *Carakasaṃhitā* and the *Suśrutasaṃhitā*. As its title suggests, it is a summary of what the author (or authors) understood to be the core contents of the older works. The *Aṣṭāṅgahṛdayasaṃhitā* is nevertheless an original work, since the choices of what constitute essential tenets and the ways these tenets are summarized, paraphrased, ordered, and brought into context with each other are testimony to the author's individual judgment and creative thought. The treatise is thought to have been composed in the beginning of the seventh century, though this again is an issue that has not been conclusively agreed on.[39] The dating of the *Aṣṭāṅgasaṃgraha* depends on its chronology relative to the *Aṣṭāṅgahṛdayasaṃhitā*, about which there has been much unresolved discussion. Accordingly, its date is also not certain.[40] The ayurvedic tradition ascribes both works to an author called Vāgbhaṭa, since this is the name given in the colophons. However, Meulenbeld (1999–2002, IA, 598) notes that the name of the author does not appear once in the main text of the *Aṣṭāṅgahṛdayasaṃhitā* and appears only in two verses in the *Aṣṭāṅgasaṃgraha* (Utt.50.203–204). Meulenbeld's conclusion is that this information is too meager to conclusively determine Vāgbhaṭa as the (single) author of either work.

Thus, the question of authorship of the medical treatises is complex and controversial. It is therefore somewhat imprecise to refer to Caraka's, Suśruta's, or Vāgbhaṭa's views on any topic instead of to "the views expressed in the *Carakasaṃhitā*", and so on.[41] However, this has become standard usage in studies on the medical treatises, and the authors' names may be understood to represent the contents of the works associated with them. This is how their names are used in this book.

In relation to the *bṛhattrayī*, the more recent works by Mādhava (c. 700 CE), Śārṅgadhara (c. 1300 CE), and Bhāvamiśra (sixteenth century CE) are categorized as the "lesser threesome" (*laghutrayī*) of Ayurveda. The idea of a greater and lesser (though still central) tradition of Ayurveda is slightly problematic, because the original use of the terms *bṛhattrayī*, *vṛddhatrayī*, and *laghutrayī* seem to have been coined at a late stage in ayurvedic history, perhaps even the nineteenth century. However, the selection of these texts to represent ayurvedic thought is not entirely random, since there are other clues that help us identify which texts are, or were, the most important ones in the tradition. For example, the importance or popularity of a text is indicated by how often its manuscripts were copied,[42] how often it is quoted in other medical works, how many commentaries on it were written, whether it was translated into other languages, and finally, whether it is still used today for ayurvedic education and practice. Jan Meulenbeld, in his landmark publication *A History of Indian Medical Literature*, provides a careful study of commentarial literature. For the *Carakasaṃhitā*, he lists more than sixty commentaries, though many of these are only available in parts as quotations in other works, or even not available at all any more (but mentioned in other works).[43] For the *Suśrutasaṃhitā*, Meulenbeld lists more than thirty commentaries,[44] and around fifty commentaries on works ascribed to Vāgbhaṭa, most of which are commentaries of the *Aṣṭāṅgahṛdayasaṃhitā*.[45] Generally, the evidence seems to point to the *Aṣṭāṅgahṛdayasaṃhitā* as having been more popular than the *Aṣṭāṅgasaṃgraha*. Meulenbeld notes that the *Aṣṭāṅgahṛdayasaṃhitā* "became the object of intensive study, as shown by the very large number of its commentaries," with important translations into Tibetan and into Persian.[46] In short, there is ample evidence for the importance of the *Carakasaṃhitā*, the *Suśrutasaṃhitā*, and the *Aṣṭāṅgahṛdayasaṃhitā* for the ayurvedic tradition. As for the *Aṣṭāṅgasaṃgraha*, one can make the argument that its importance lies in its link to the *Aṣṭāṅgahṛdayasaṃhitā*, though there are very few manuscripts of it. Despite there being little evidence of its importance in ayurvedic history, it is used as part of the government-approved syllabus in ayurvedic universities and colleges in India.

In the case of the *Mādhavanidāna* (which is referred to as the *Rogaviniścaya* by the author himself),[47] Meulenbeld cites numerous references to and quotations from it and notes that many later works draw heavily on it without specifying it as a source. About twenty-four commentaries on it exist.[48] The *Śārṅgadharasaṃhitā*'s popularity, on the other hand, cannot be deduced from the number of commentaries on it: there are only three.[49] Nevertheless, it is one of the most enduringly popular ayurvedic texts, which is evident from the "scores of handwritten copies" found in almost every manuscript library across India today.[50] Recipes from the *Śārṅgadharasaṃhitā* are still used by the modern ayurvedic pharmaceutical industry. Finally, the *Bhāvaprakāśa*'s popularity is attested through its many manuscript copies and the many references made to it in other medical works.[51] All of these works form part of the curriculum of government-approved ayurvedic education in India today.

I have included extracts from one further ayurvedic treatise in this study, namely the *Kāśyapasaṃhitā*, a medical manual on pediatrics that dates to around the seventh century CE. This treatise has not had the same importance for the ayurvedic tradition as those described above. However, it is an early text that offers additional, and sometimes differing viewpoints to the classic treatises and thus provides a more complete picture of the early ayurvedic Weltanschauung.

The *Kāśyapasaṃhitā* has come down to us in two manuscripts, one of which contains only a small portion of the text, and the second of which, though much more extensive, is damaged and incomplete as well. The editions of the *Kāśyapasaṃhitā* are based on the second manuscript.[52] The *Kāśyapasaṃhitā* that has been preserved seems to be the revised version of an older treatise. While Kaśyapa (not Kāśyapa) is the original author, Vātsya is named as the reviser of the treatise, and the text that he rewrote may have been called the *Vṛddhajīvakīyatantra* (this title is found in some of the colophons of the manuscripts of the *Kāśyapasaṃhitā*). Meulenbeld (1999–2002, IIA, 40–41) notes that due to the editorial work by Vātsya, "the sections of the *Kāśyapasaṃhitā* from the Sūtrasthāna up to the Kalpasthāna consist of two layers which can, unfortunately, not be distinguished from each other." Its dating to the seventh century relies on the fact that it has some nosological features not yet found in the *Carakasaṃhitā*, the *Suśrutasaṃhitā*, or the *Aṣṭāṅgahṛdayasaṃhitā*, but which appear in the *Mādhavanidāna*. At the same time, Kaśyapa's description of the diseases differs substantially from Mādhava's, so that the assumption is that Mādhava's text was unknown to him (or not yet an influential text). This places Kaśyapa's text into either the same period as Mādhava's treatise or a somewhat earlier period, that is, around the seventh century CE.

Two further medical treatises that I mention, but do not cite extensively in this study are the *Bhelasaṃhitā* and the *Hārītasaṃhitā*. The *Bhelasaṃhitā*, a treatise on internal medicine (*kāyacikitsā*), has come down to us in one incomplete and faulty manuscript, kept at the Sarasvatī Mahāl Library in Tanjore, and one further fragment of a paper manuscript discovered in Central Asia. The extant editions of the *Bhelasaṃhitā* are based on the Tanjore manuscript. The *Bhelasaṃhitā* is often quoted in other medical works, but many of these quotations cannot be found in the version of the *Bhelasaṃhitā* that has been preserved in the Tanjore manuscript. The text of the *Bhelasaṃhitā* as we know it contains reference to the *Carakasaṃhitā*, so that we can assume the *Bhelasaṃhitā* came later. It also has parallels with the *Suśrutasaṃhitā*, which may mean either that it derived its parallel contents from the *Suśrutasaṃhitā* or that both texts had a common source, or depended on the same floating tradition of medicine. It is mentioned in the Bower manuscript, and reference to recipes from it are found in both the *Aṣṭāṅgasaṃgraha* and the *Aṣṭāṅgahṛdayasaṃhitā*. Meulenbeld (1999–2002, IIA, 24), however, concludes that the evidence taken together points to "a period after Vāgbhaṭa, about the seventh century or somewhat later, as the age that saw the completion of the text of the *Bhelasaṃhitā* represented by the Tanjore MS."

The *Hārītasaṃhitā* is a textbook that deals principally with internal medicine (*kāyacikitsā*). It is written in the form of a dialogue between Hārīta and Ātreya (the same sage-teacher who also teaches Agniveśa in the *Carakasaṃhitā* and Bhela in the *Bhelasaṃhitā*), and its colophons correspondingly give it the title of *Ātreyabhāṣita Hārītottara* (but also, once, *Vaidyasarvasva*). Despite this veneer of antiquity, it was probably written between 700–1000 CE, according to Meulenbeld (1999–2002, IIA, 60).

The Commentaries

The commentaries on the medical classics can help us understand the meaning of passages that are not immediately clear to a modern reader. Often, however, one finds that unclear passages, or opaque parts within them, are not explained by the commentator at all, while other details that seem rather obvious are expounded on at length. At the same time, it is in the commentaries that we sometimes find a meta discussion of topics that is lacking in the classics themselves.

As noted, we know of about sixty commentaries on the *Carakasaṃhitā*. Most of these are lost, and we only know of them through quotations or references to them in other works. Others are preserved in fragments, such as the *Carakanyāsa*, of Haricandra (or Hariścandra, or Bhaṭṭāra(ka)hari(ś)candra) or Jejjaṭa's *Nirantarapadavyākhyā*. The main early commentary that has been preserved and is available to us today is Cakrapāṇidatta's *Āyurvedadīpikā*, written in Bengal during the eleventh century CE. This is the commentary I have consulted for this study. Much later commentaries include Gaṅgādhara Kavirāja's *Jalpakalpataru*, written in the early nineteenth century, and Yogīndranāthasena's *Carakopaskāra*, written in the late nineteenth century.

We also know of a large number of commentaries on the *Suśrutasaṃhitā* through references to them or quotations from them. The earliest one to have been preserved, albeit only in parts, is Cakrapāṇidatta's *Bhānumatī*, of which we have the section that deals with the Sūtrasthāna. The more complete *Nibandhasaṃgraha*, by Ḍalhaṇa, was written in about the twelfth century CE, as established by the fact that Ḍalhaṇa quotes Cakrapāṇidatta and is in turn quoted by Hemādri (c. thirteenth century CE).[53] This is the commentary used here. In addition, a partly preserved commentary by Jejjaṭa (the title of which is unknown) is extensively quoted in Ḍalhaṇa's commentary. I discuss one such quotation in chapter 6. A modern commentary on the *Suśrutasaṃhitā* by Hārāṇacandra, who lived in the late nineteenth and early twentieth centuries, also exists, called the *Suśrutārthasaṃdīpana*.

Several commentaries of the *Aṣṭāṅgahṛdayasaṃhitā* have been at least partly preserved, and as in the case of the *Carakasaṃhitā* and the *Suśrutasaṃhitā*, we know of several more through references to or quotations from them. The *Padārthacandrikā* by Candranandana, which was written between the eighth and the eleventh centuries, according to Meulenbeld (1999–2002, IA, 663) is one of the early commentaries. Only a small portion of this work has been edited, though parts of it can also be found in notes to the edition of the *Aṣṭāṅgahṛdayasaṃhitā* by Kuṃṭe et al. (1995). It is also quoted extensively in Aruṇadatta's commentary on the *Aṣṭāṅgahṛdayasaṃhitā*, the *Sarvāṅgasundarā*, which was probably written in the latter half of the twelfth century. This commentary, Hemādri's commentary *Āyurvedarasāyana* (probably written in the late thirteenth century), and Indu's *Śaśilekhā* (probably written in the latter half of the twelfth century, though the Indian tradition claims that Indu was a direct pupil of Vāgbhaṭa)[54] were consulted for this study. Indu also wrote a commentary on the *Aṣṭāṅgasaṃgraha*, also entitled *Śaśilekhā*. However, neither this commentary nor another on the *Aṣṭāṅgasaṃgraha* was available to me.

There are three known commentaries on the *Śārṅgadharasaṃhitā*: Āḍhamalla's *Pradīpikā* (or *Śārṅgadharadīpikā* according to the colophons), Kāśīrāma's *Gūḍhārthadīpikā*, and Rudrabhaṭṭa's (or Rudradharabhaṭṭa's) *Āyurvedadīpikā* (or *Gūḍhāntadīpikā*). These date to possibly the fourteenth century, either the sixteenth or seventeenth century, and the late sixteenth/early seventeenth centuries, respectively.[55] We do not know of any commentaries on the *Kāśyapasaṃhitā*. Finally, there is one Sanskrit commentary on the *Bhāvaprakāśa*: the *Śrīraṇavīrasiṃhadevāvalokanasadvaidyasiddhāntaratnākara* by Jayadeva, which was written in the late nineteenth century. This commentary was not available to me. However, the edition by Srikantha Murthy (1998–) contains a Hindi commentary called "Vidyotinī" that I have consulted.

Other Source Texts

I use a number of texts in this study for a comparison with the ayurvedic treatises. Among the most important of these is the *Kauṭilīya Arthaśāstra*, an ancient Indian treatise on statecraft, economic policy, and military strategy ascribed to the author Kauṭilya (or Kauṭalya). As is so often the case with ancient Indian texts, the date of the *Kauṭilīya Arthaśāstra* is not entirely certain. According to Trautmann (1971, 167–187), it is a composition from no earlier than the second century CE, but based on earlier material. The *Arthaśāstra* is an early source on how physicians and their work were dealt with as part of a state structure, and provides us with some answers to questions regarding physicians' livelihood and their place in society that remain open on reading the medical treatises. We find some references to this work (or, at least, to an *Arthaśāstra*) in the medical treatises that attest to some connection between them.[56]

There are also parallels with Buddhist literature in the ayurvedic treatises, which have been discussed in some length by Zysk (1998 [1991]). The Pāli Canon is one text source with materials that correspond to passages in the medical treatises. Written in Pāli, the Canon is the standard collection of scriptures of the Theravada ("the teaching of the elders") Buddhist tradition. This tradition holds that the Canon was composed in North India and preserved orally until it was committed to writing in the first century BCE. The *Mahāvagga*, which I mention a number of times in this study, belongs to the Pāli Canon's Vinayapiṭaka, the section on monastic rules for monks and nuns. There is also some relevant material in the Suttanipāta and in the Aṅguttaranikāya, which are both part of the Pāli Canon's Suttapiṭaka (the section on teachings), and again in the Pacittiya (the section on rules entailing confession), which is part of the Vinayapiṭaka.

Further similarities are found with Buddhaghosa's *Visuddhimagga* ("the path to purity"). Written in the fifth century CE, it is considered the most important Theravada text outside the Pāli Canon. A discussion of the concepts of kindness (*maitrī*) and compassion (*karuṇā*) in the *Visuddhimagga* is paralleled by Caraka's description of the characteristics of a good physician in Sū.9.26. In addition, a parallel passage on the concepts of kindness and compassion has similar wording to that of the *Visuddhimagga* in the *Pātañjala Yogasūtra* (1.33). The date of this foundational work on Yoga philosophy is uncertain, and depends to some extent on whether one assumes its commentary, the *Bhāṣya*, to have been written simultaneously with the main corpus by Patañjali, or separately, by another author. Philipp Maas (2006, 16) judges it likely that both the main text and commentary were written by the same author and concludes that they were probably written between 325 and 425 CE.

Some material in brahmanic religious law (*dharma*) literature is closely linked with passages in the medical treatises. The genre of *dharma* literature encompasses a number of works, the best known of which is the Law Code of Manu, the *Mānavadharmaśāstra*, also known as the *Manusmṛti* (c. second century CE).[57] Manu's legal code was preceded by the *dharmasūtras* (legal works written in aphoristic prose) of Āpastamba, Gautama, Baudhāyana, and Vasiṣṭha.[58] These works deal with ritual activities and issues concerning moral conduct and are principally addressed to persons belonging to the brahmin, or priest classes, but also to those of the ruling classes (*kṣatriya*) and the trade classes (*vaiśya*). Another class of literature, the *gṛhyasūtras*, deals specifically with the domestic ceremonies and rituals of the "twice-born" (*dvija*, members of priest, ruling, and trade classes who underwent an rite regarded as their second birth). Both *dharmasūtras* and *gṛhyasūtras* are part of the body of literature collectively called *kalpasūtra* (rules concerning ritual), which is one of the six Vedāṅgas (auxiliary disciplines for the understanding of the Vedas).

Structure

This study is divided into a main part and appendices that correspond to the chapters of the main part. The main part discusses the topics listed in this introduction: the roles of the persons involved in medicine, their relationships with each other, and the moral underpinnings of their exchanges. The discussion is based on the analysis of relevant text sections from the selected classical treatises. The translations of these text passages are embedded in my discussion; the Sanskrit texts of the selected passages are given in the corresponding appendices. The appendices broadly follow the order of sequence in which the texts chosen for discussion or analysis appear in the main part of the book. If a translated passage is part of a larger section that is quoted in another chapter, the Sanskrit text of the short passage will be found as part of the larger section. The Sanskrit text of passages from commentarial literature are given in the notes. Unless indicated otherwise, all translations are my own.

Texts and Translations

For the text of the *Carakasaṃhitā*, I have mainly used the fifth edition by Trikamji Acarya (1992a), which includes the text of Cakrapāṇidatta's *Āyurveda-dīpikā*. However, for passages from the Vimānasthāna, I have also consulted the critical edition of the Vimānasthāna of the *Carakasaṃhitā* that was prepared by the Vienna project under Karin Preisendanz.[59] At the time this study was written, the critical edition was still a work in progress, but Vimānasthāna 8.13–14, a key passage on medical ethics, had been completed. I have also consulted the Sanskrit text and English translation by Sharma (2003), and have used translations of text passages from the *Carakasaṃhitā* by Wujastyk (2003) and Selby (2005).

For the text of the *Suśrutasaṃhitā*, I have used the edition by Trikamji Acarya (1992b), which includes Ḍalhaṇa's *Nibandhasaṃgraha* and Gayadāsācārya's commentary on the Nidānasthāna, the *Nyāyacandrikā*. I have also consulted the text and translation by Sharma (1999–2001) and have used translations of text passages from the *Suśrutasaṃhitā* by Wujastyk (2003).

For the *Aṣṭāṅgahṛdayasaṃhitā*, I have used the edition by Kuṃṭe et al. (1995), which includes the commentary by Aruṇadatta, the *Sarvāṅgasundarā*, and the commentary by Hemādri, the *Āyurvedarasāyana*. I have also consulted the text and translation by Srikantha Murthy (1991–95), as well as the German translation by Hilgenberg and Kirfel (1941). For the *Aṣṭāṅgasaṃgraha*, I have used the edition by Srikantha Murthy (1995–97).

For the *Śārṅgadharasaṃhitā*, I have used the edition by Vidyasagar (1986), which includes Āḍhamalla's *Dīpikā* and Kāśīrāma's *Gūḍārthadīpikā*. I have used the edition by Srikantha Murthy (1993) and the translation of the first ten chapters by Meulenbeld (1974) for the *Mādhavanidāna*, the edition by Srikantha Murthy (1998–) for the *Bhāvaprakāśa*, the edition by Tewari (1996) for the *Kāśyapasaṃhitā*, and finally the edition of Krishnamurthy (2000) for the *Bhelasaṃhitā*.

A very substantial collection of Sanskrit texts has been typed into machine-readable format by Vedic Engineering, including the *Carakasaṃhitā*, the *Suśrutasaṃhitā*, the *Aṣṭāṅgahṛdayasaṃhitā*, the *Aṣṭāṅgasaṃgraha*, the

Śārṅgadharasaṃhitā, the *Mādhavanidāna*, and the *Bhāvaprakāśa*.[60] I have used these extensively for key-term searches.

Technical Terms

I was relieved to find only few plant names in the text passages chosen for this study, since plant identification is one of the greater problems in the translation of ayurvedic texts.[61] In the few cases in which plant names occur in the selected passages, I have tried to identify them using the online plant database of the Foundation for the Revitalization of Local Health Traditions (FRLHT), which gives the Latin nomenclature for Sanskrit plant names, as well as Sanskrit and vernacular synonyms (see www.frlht.org.in/meta).[62] I have in some cases used the website zipcodezoo.com, whose primary data provider is the Global Biodiversity Information Facility (GBIF), to match the Latin names with English ones if they are not given on the FRLHT site. This method is not failsafe, since a Sanskrit term search on the FRLHT database usually brings up a number of possibilities, any of which could be the plant in question. I have further consulted the encyclopedias by Griffiths (1994), Warrier et al. (1994–96), Nadkarni (1954), and Sivarajan and Balachandran (1994). Nevertheless, some doubt remains regarding the correct identification of some of the named plants.

1

The Pillars of Treatment

THE INDIAN CLASSICAL medical treatises identify four agents or constituents of medicine in a standard formula: the physician, the medicine, the attendant, and the patient. Together they form the "four pillars," or "quartet of pillars" (*catuṣpāda*, or *pādacatuṣṭaya*), of treatment.[63]

In definitions of the four pillars, we learn about the qualities desired in each, their relations to each other, and their respective places within medical hierarchy. Definitions of medical treatment as consisting of four pillars are found in nearly all of the oldest classical medical texts—the *Carakasaṃhitā*, the *Suśrutasaṃhitā*, the *Aṣṭāṅgasaṃgraha*, the *Aṣṭāṅgahṛdayasaṃhitā*, the *Kāśyapasaṃhitā*, and the *Bhelasaṃhitā*.[64] The youngest of the classical medical texts, the *Bhāvaprakāśa* (Pūrv.6.37) describes seven components (*aṅga*) rather than four pillars.

I will introduce the passages in the medical treatises that describe the pillars of medical treatment, discussing their setting within their respective treatises and comparing each treatise's treatment of the subject with that of the others.

I will then outline the treatises' definitions of three of the four pillars, namely the physician, the patient, and the attendant, and supplement these definitions with further ones from other parts of the medical compendia. Since this study focuses on human actions and relationships within a medical setting, the fourth pillar of treatment, medicine, will not be discussed separately. Though medical plants and substances, their medicinal properties, preparations, and uses are described at length throughout the ayurvedic compendia (and probably form the largest part of these), the ethics of their use is confined to few statements regarding the care a physician must take in utilizing them. This care concerns the correct use of medicines in terms of choice of drug and dosage to achieve the patient's cure, and to avoid harming the patient through inappropriate medication. There is no indication of any specific care being directed toward the plants themselves (as, for example, through practices of sustainable harvesting) that would point to an ecological ethic.

My discussion of how physicians are represented by the medical authors also includes their representations of the good physician's antithesis—the quack, who features both in Caraka's four-pillar definition and in other passages.

Finally, the category of attendant is widened to include other persons who contribute in various ways to medical practice, such as wet-nurses, kitchen staff, and persons who provide requisite knowledge about plant materials.

Definitions of the pillars of treatment

The Four Pillars of Treatment According to Caraka

Carakasaṃhitā Sūtrasthāna 9:

"Now I shall give a brief lesson on the four pillars," said Lord Ātreya. (1–2) The physician, the medicine, the attendant and the patient are the quartet of pillars, which, when it is endowed with good qualities, should be known as the means to the calming of disorders. (3) The imbalance of the humors is regarded as a disorder, their equilibrium as their natural state.[65] Health is known as ease, and illness as disease. (4) Medical practice is considered to be the activity of the praised four,[66] the physician etc., which is directed at the equilibrium of the humors when there is a disorder of the humors. (5) A thorough knowledge of the discipline, extensive observation of practice, skill, and cleanliness: These should be known as the quartet of good qualities in a physician. (6) Plentifulness, suitability,[67] having various preparations,[68] and excellent quality are regarded as the quartet of good qualities in medicines.[69] (7) Knowledge of attendance, skill, affection for [his] master, and cleanliness: That is the quartet of qualities in an attendant. (8) Mindfulness, obedience, fearlessness, and, moreover, providing information on the diseases are thought to be the qualities of the patient. (9) The four pillars, consisting of sixteen qualities, are the means to success, but the physician who has knowledge, who governs, and who applies effort is the most important amongst these.[70] (10) Just as pot, fuel, and fire are the cook's means to cooking, and land, army, and weapons the conqueror's means to conquest, the pillars, beginning with the patient, are called the physician's means to success. Therefore the physician is the most important means in medicine. (11–12) Like clay, stick, potter's wheel, thread, etc. without a potter, the three pillars without the physician do not produce results.[71] (13) Even though there are three [other] pillars, it is the knowledgeable and the ignorant physician that are the reason that terrible disorders

> disappear like the city of *gandharvas*,[72] and that others, waiting for quick remedy, grow. (14–15ab) It is better to burn oneself than to be administered medicine by one who is ignorant. (15cd) Fearful, because of employing his hands like a blind person, and because of his ignorance, the ignorant physician goes about treatment like a boat controlled by the wind. (16) One who, by chance having assisted one whose duration of life was fixed, believes himself a physician, directly kills hundreds whose duration of life isn't fixed.[73] (17) Therefore, a physician who is engaged in the set of four: the discipline, comprehension of its meaning, its application, and the observation of medical practice is called a 'saver of life.' (18) One who has the fourfold knowledge of cause, symptom, cure, and prevention of diseases is the best physician and fit for a king.[74] (19) A weapon, learning, and water depend on their recipient to manifest their merits and defects; therefore [the physician] should improve his knowledge for the sake of medicine. (20) Knowledge, reason, understanding, mindfulness, devotion, and action: nothing is unattainable for one who has these six qualities. (21) Knowledge, intelligence, observation of treatment, practice, accomplishment, and support:[75] even only one of these is sufficient for obtaining the title 'physician.' (22) One who has all these splendid qualities of knowledge, etc., truly deserves the title 'physician' and gives happiness to living beings. (23) The science[76] is a light that has the purpose of illuminating, [and] one's intelligence is that which perceives. A physician who undertakes treatment with both harmoniously joined cannot do wrong. (24) Because the three [other] pillars rely on the physician in medical treatment, the physician should put persevering effort into the perfection of his qualities. (25) Kindness and compassion for those who are ill, affection for the remediable, and equanimity toward those in their natural state, this is the quartet of a physician's conduct."[77] (26)

Caraka devotes an entire chapter to the subject of the four pillars, placing it in the Sūtrasthāna, the section on the fundamentals of medicine. The location of the chapter in the Sūtrasthāna gives its contents the status of foundational knowledge on medicine. However, the topic of the four pillars is not elaborated in later parts of the work (as many of the other subjects introduced in the Sūtrasthāna are) and thus is probably intended to contextualize the use of medicine rather than to serve as prerequisite knowledge for actual medical practice.

The position of this chapter, the ninth within the Sūtrasthāna, is worth noting. It is preceded by a chapter dedicated to the sense organs, which ends with a section on good conduct (*sadvṛtta*). Good conduct here is depicted as equivalent to a healthy lifestyle, in that it is understood to prevent the derangement of the sense organs, and thus to forestall the arising of illness.[78] This chapter therefore describes a nonmedical situation, in which there is no patient (and therefore no doctor, medicine, or attendant), but a person with responsibility for his own well-being and indeed the agency to maintain his good health and to prevent illness. This is broadly also the general theme in the preceding chapters (Ca.Sū.5–7). Chapter 9 thus represents a shift in content from the more widely ranging "knowledge of life" to its more narrowly circumscribed subcategory of medicine (*cikitsā*).

A brief overview of chapter 9 reveals the following structure: After the introductory sentences, the chapter's treatment of the topic begins in verse 3 with the definition of the four pillars as the means to calming disorders (*vikāravyupaśānti*). This is followed up in verse 4 by a definition of disorder, and conversely, of the natural state: health. Verse 5 concludes that medicine (*cikitsā*) is the employment of the four pillars against disorders. The following verses (6–9) give the desired qualities of the pillars, with one verse dedicated to each. Verses 10–15 explain why the physician is the most important among the four pillars. Verses 15–17 deal with quacks; the rest of the chapter is again dedicated to the good physician and his qualities. Verse 18 offers an alternative (albeit similar) set of four qualities to the initial four proposed in verse 6. Verse 19 warns that a physician must practice his knowledge and hone his skills. Two more sets of six qualities are added in verses 21–23 (though those given in 21 could be understood to describe universal positive attributes rather than ones specific to a good physician); and a final set of four qualities closes the topic in verse 26. Verses 27–28 summarize the contents of the chapter.

What becomes clear immediately from this summary is that the majority of verses are dedicated to the physician. The two sets of four and two sets of six qualities that lay out the characteristics of a good physician add up to about twenty distinct qualities, due to some overlap (see table 1a and b).[79]

Table 1a

Verse 6 *śrute paryavadātatva, bahuśo dṛṣṭakarmatā, dākṣya, śauca*
Verse 18 *śāstra, arthajñāna, pravṛtti, karmadarśana*
Verse 21 *vidyā, vitarka, vijñāna, smṛti, tatparatā, kriyā*
Verse 22 *vidyā, mati, karmadṛṣṭi, abhyāsa, siddhi, āśraya*
Verse 26 *(ārteṣu) maitrī, kāruṇya, (śakye) prīti, (prakṛtistheṣu) upekṣaṇa*

Table 1b

Verse 6 accomplishment in the discipline, extensive observation of practice, skill, cleanliness

Verse 18 [knowledge of the] discipline, comprehension of meaning, application, observation of medical practice
Verse 21 knowledge, reason, understanding, mindfulness, devotion, action
Verse 22 knowledge, intelligence, observation of treatment, practice, accomplishment, support
Verse 26 kindness, compassion (to the ill), affection (to the remediable), indifference (to the healthy)

Most of these characteristics belong to the semantic field of cognition: knowledge, reason, understanding, intelligence, and mindfulness. Experience is also given a prominent role, with key words such as skill (*dākṣya*), application (*pravṛtti*), therapeutic action (*kriyā*), and practice (*abhyāsa*). The terms *dṛṣṭakarmatā*, *karmadarśana*, and *karmadṛṣṭi* also belong to the category of experience. I understand these to refer to having witnessed practice. For example, I have translated *dṛṣṭakarmatā* in verse 6 as "observation of practice." However, it could also be translated as "the state of being one whose actions are seen or proved" or "the state of being one tried by practice"—in other words, it could refer to having practical experience rather than to having witnessed practice. In any case, both witnessing practice and the actual application of practice constitute experience, and are part of a process of acquiring knowledge and skill.

One notable grammatical characteristic of Caraka's delineation of the four pillars of medicine is the almost complete lack of the use of the optative or imperative mode, or of gerundives.[80] A physician as one of the four pillars of medicine *is* skilled, rather than *ought to be* skilled. The parallel passages in the other medical works concur in their use of verbal mood. Thus, we are confronted with the fundamental question of whether the descriptions of the four pillars represent an ethical evaluation of good or bad medical practice or merely function as a neutral description of "what is." Caraka's text never specifically qualifies the physician (or patient or attendant) as "good" or "bad." We do, however, find some instances of value judgment: Verse 12 describes the four pillars of treatment as the "means to success" (*siddhau kāraṇa*). Verse 19 speaks of the "best physician" (*bhiṣaktama*) who is "fit for a king" (*rājārha*), and verse 23 indicates that the title "physician" (*vaidya*) is one that is deserved or earned by one with particular qualities. Further distinction is made between a knowledgeable and an ignorant physician, the former giving relief to patients, the latter causing havoc and death. Verse 15 is unequivocal in stating that it would be better to burn oneself than to submit to an ignorant physician's ministrations. All of this amounts to quite a substantial number of value judgments, so we can safely conclude that Caraka's definition of the four pillars does indeed represent an ethic of good (and bad) medical practice.

Note that in this list of judgments, only very few items are concerned with the doctor–patient relationship. Only in verse 26—the last in the section—is a physician's attitude to the patient touched on with keywords such as kindness (*maitrī*), compassion (*kāruṇya*), and affection (*prīti*) but also indifference (or detachment: *upekṣaṇa*). These concepts are very similar to the four "divine states" known in Buddhism, the *brahmavihāra:*[81] *mettā, karuṇā, muditā,* and *upekkhā,* as laid out in the Pāli Canon's Brahmavihārasutta (Suttapiṭaka, Aṅguttaranikāya 10.208),[82] and, in more detail, in Buddhaghosa's Visuddhimagga 9.[83] A further parallel exists with Yogasūtra 1.33, in which the attitudes of kindness (*maitrī*) to the happy, compassion (*karuṇa*) with the unhappy, joy (*muditā*) in regard to the virtuous, and detachment (*upekṣā*) in regard to those without virtue are described as the cause of clarity of the mind.[84] The position of these concepts at the very end of Sūtrasthāna 9, and the fact that they are the only injunctions regarding the physician's attitude to his patient, make them seem an afterthought rather than a core definition of the good physician's characteristics. We are left with the impression that the main requirement of the physician does not concern the quality of his relationship with the patient, but rather his knowledge and skill. This is also broadly how Suśruta presents his account of the physician as one of the four pillars, as we will see from the following.

The Four Pillars of Treatment According to Suśruta

Suśrutasaṃhitā Sūtrasthāna 34.15cd–24

The physician, the one afflicted by illness, the medicine, and the attendant—these are the pillars of medicine, the means to cure. (15cd–16ab) By means of the three [other] excellent pillars, the fourth, an excellent physician can cure even a serious illness within a short time. But without the physician, the three [other] pillars, even if they are excellent, are useless, just as the Udgātṛ, the Hotṛ, and the Brahman are useless at a sacrifice without the Adhvaryu.[85] (16cd–18ab) But an excellent physician can always rescue a patient on his own, as a helmsman can rescue a boat in the sea without oarsmen. (18cd–19ab) The physician who has accurately studied the meaning of the teachings, has observed practice and practiced himself, who is light-handed, clean, and strong, equipped with instruments and drugs, confident, sensible, determined, and skilled, honest, and pious is known as a

> pillar (of treatment). (19cd–21ab) A patient who is long-lived, resolute, curable, wealthy, and also prudent, pious, and attentive to what the doctor says is known as a pillar [of treatment]. (21cd–22ab) A medicine grown in a suitable place and harvested on a suitable day, in appropriate quantities, with an agreeable smell, color, and taste, removing [excess] humors,[86] not producing sickness, harmless when wrongly used, and administered after close examination and on time is known as a pillar [of treatment]. (22cd–23) A loving assistant who is not squeamish and strong, who is ready to care for the sick, follows the physician's orders, and is unwearying is thought of as a pillar [of treatment]. (24)

Suśruta places his description of the four pillars of treatment in the second half of a chapter on military medicine in the Sūtrasthāna (chapter 34, 15–end). The description is a non sequitur to Suśruta's preceding explanations of why a physician should be part of a military campaign and what his role would be on the battlefield (i.e., to protect the king). In the context of military medicine, the agents are the king, the physician, and the priest rather than the physician, the patient, the medicine, and the attendant. Note that this is the only instance in the ayurvedic treatises (which give very little information on a physician's place in society) in which the physician's position is fairly clearly defined: he is part of the military campaign and accountable to the king and the priest.

While the transition from military medicine to more general medicine is abrupt, and the description of the four pillars could easily form an independent chapter, the two sections share a common element: they outline hierarchies. In the first section, the physician is at the bottom of the ranking system: he is subordinate to the priest, and both he and the priest are subservient to the king. In the second, the physician is at the top of the ranking order. The priest is not featured as one of the pillars, and the king—the patient par excellence according to Zimmermann[87]—is replaced by the common patient, who is not accorded the same exalted position. Suśruta makes much of the physician's eminence among the pillars: four verses out of ten are dedicated to this theme. His list of the pillars' characteristics is similar in content to Caraka's, but he does not follow Caraka's scheme of four characteristics each, and he changes Caraka's sequence from physician, medicine, attendant, and patient to physician, patient, medicine, and attendant. The most striking difference in Suśruta's list of the physician's characteristics is his emphasis on physical abilities, particularly light-handedness, swiftness, and strength, and their psychological counterparts, readiness of mind and resolve. This probably reflects the specific medical context Suśruta envisages, that is, surgery (as opposed to general medical treatment), which would indeed require such qualities, particularly in view of the unavailability (or lack of knowledge) of anaesthetics. Suśruta does not give any comment on the emotional link between doctor and patient, omitting any parallel statement to Caraka's injunction of kindness and compassion toward the patient. The relationship between doctor and patient is reduced to a one-way obligation of the patient to the physician in which the patient must be "attentive" to the physician. Verse 24 gives a glimpse into what might have been the closer relationship in the medical process: that between the attendant and the patient. Suśruta's attendant is required to be friendly and accepting and, significantly, to be ready to care for the sick. This is an important point to make in a society organized on principles of class distinction that are at least partly based on claims of a person's hereditary and/or acquired status of purity. An attendant's job would have required contact with the patient, regardless of both the patient's status and his own.[88] This could have had implications for both the patient and the attendant. Nursing would also have involved contact with impure substances, like blood and feces, which would very likely have been problematic. This raises the question of the medical attendant's status within society. Who would have been willing to do this work and at the same time have been acceptable to the patients? Unfortunately, Suśruta does not provide any answer to these questions here or elsewhere in his compendium. We will, however, return to this question later.

The Four Pillars of Treatment According to Vāgbhaṭa

Aṣṭāṅgahṛdayasaṃhitā Sūtrasthāna 1.27–29 *and Aṣṭāṅgasaṃgraha Sūtrasthāna* 2.21–25ab

> The physician, the medicines, the attendant, and the patient are called the quartet of pillars of medical treatment. Each one has four qualities. (27) The physician is skilled, has received the meaning of the teachings from a preceptor, has witnessed practice, and is clean. The medicine has numerous preparations and many qualities, is palatable and suitable. (28) The attendant is affectionate, clean, able, and intelligent. The patient is wealthy, obedient to the physician, provides information,[89] and is resolute. (29)

The *Aṣṭāṅgahṛdayasaṃhitā* and the *Aṣṭāṅgasaṃgraha* give identical accounts of the four pillars of medicine in Sū.1.27–29 and Sū.2.21–25ab, respectively. Their short summaries of the four pillars of medicine follow Caraka's sequence: physician, medicine, attendant, patient. They reiterate Caraka's initial division into four characteristics for each pillar and share a number of items of his list of characteristics. We also find, however, some keywords from Suśruta's definition, as well as a number of characteristics that are not quoted from either Caraka or Suśruta. One interesting difference between Vāgbhaṭa's versions and Caraka's is the use of the term *tīrthātta-śāstrārtha*—"who has received the teachings from a preceptor," which stands in lieu of Caraka's *śrute paryavadātatva*—"thorough knowledge of the tradition." It has a parallel in Suśruta's *tattvādhigataśāstrārtha*—"who has truly learnt the meaning of the teachings."[90] However, whether we read *tattvādhigataśāstrārtha* or *tīrthāttaśāstrārtha*, the point is that the teachings of medicine are to be learnt or received in a particular way in order to enable the physician to fully understand medicine. This, first, confirms the importance of a physician's knowledge of medicine as a prerequisite to his practice: his knowledge gives him the authority to practice. Second, it suggests a different aspect of what gives a physician authority or authorization: his connection with a venerated teacher, and thus with an authoritative teaching. As Cakrapāṇidatta suggested, this may be what Caraka meant with his mention of "support" (*āśraya*) as one of the qualifications to being called a *vaidya*.[91] The question of lineage is also taken up by Kaśyapa as one of his first points on what establishes a physician as accomplished.

The Four Pillars of Treatment According to Kaśyapa

Kāśyapasaṃhitā Sūtrasthāna 26.3–11

> I will explain the means by which the perfection of medical treatment is arrived at.[92] There are four pillars of medicine. If these, namely the physician, the medicine, the patient and the attendant, are possessed of good qualities, a curable disease cannot prevail. (3) The physician, then, has a good teacher,[93] has properly received Vedic knowledge, is discerning, has often witnessed medical treatments, has knowledge of efficacious compounds, is able, competent, clean, and modestly dressed, has friendly relations with all beings, is successful, displays religious merit and wealth, delights in truth, compassion, generosity, and propriety, honors and follows the gods, the twice-born, teachers, and accomplished persons, becomes increasingly competent in procedures, is deferential to teachers and elders, adheres to logic [*nyāya*], is free from fear, greed, delusion, anger, and falsehood, does not slander, is not eager for alcohol, is handsome, and is free from evil practices. (4) Perfection in a medicine, then, is having grown in a good place, and having been harvested on time, and having been produced on time, being unspoilt, being free from damage by fire, water, insects, feces, urine,

age, etc., being useful for various illnesses, and being administered gradually and according to rule. (5)

Perfection in a patient, then, is [having] a curable disease, stability of nature, strength, mind, body, sense-organs, will, and vital power, [giving] exact communication of causes, early symptoms, pain, complications, development, and suitable and nonsuitable medication, (having) faith in the wet-nurse, respect to gods, brahmins, teachers, physicians, medicines, and friends, piousness, good behavior, doing as told, and self-command.[94] (6)

Perfection in an attendant, then, is the ability to prepare decoctions, health, strength, devotion to his master, knowledge of medical practice, skill, cleanliness, quick action, experience in all treatments, unsqueamishness, not having low family relations, straightforwardness, self-command, having conquered anger etc., and patience. (7)

On this, there are the verses:
Some believe the patient to be the most important of this set of four pillars, since it is for his sake that the other three pillars are desired to be full of merit here. (8)
"That is not so," said Prajāpati: "The physician is the foundation of medicine, since the three [others] are under the control of the physician, and success also rests upon the physician. (9)
With the eye of knowledge he plans, performs, and directs. Therefore, a physician who is endowed with knowledge and discernment is the most important [of the pillars]. (10)
When, Jīvaka, the four pillars are perfect, the physician becomes entitled to religious merit, wealth, and fame."(11)

Kaśyapa devotes all of chapter 26 of the Sūtrasthāna to his definition of the four pillars of medicine. The chapter is written in a mix of prose and verse, with the part in prose (3–7) covering the four pillars' characteristics and the part in verse (8–10) giving a discussion of the hierarchy between the pillars. His list of the four pillars' characteristics is extensive, suggesting no less than twenty-two requirements of the physician, seven of the medicine, nine of the patient, and fifteen of the attendant. Verses 8–10 are presented as quotations, the source of which is not given.

Kaśyapa's version mostly develops further the themes already introduced by Caraka and Suśruta, with no major deviations from points they give attention to. The physician that Kaśyapa envisages seems to be of high social standing. He is wealthy and well educated: versed not only in diverse aspects of medicine but also in Vedic scriptures, as well as in logic (*nyāya*). Kaśyapa's checklist contains more items concerning the physician's etiquette—the prescribed limits of appropriate social behavior within a set situation—than the other authors offer in their four-pillar definitions.

Kaśyapa's description of the perfect patient elaborates on one subject that is only touched on very briefly by Caraka and Vāgbhaṭa (and not mentioned by Suśruta at all): the idea that the patient should give the physician full and clear information on his state of being. Kaśyapa also suggests that the patient should have faith in the wet-nurse. This requirement is specific to the obstetric context of Kaśyapa's work and is not featured in any of the other treatises.

The Components of Treatment According to Bhāvamiśra

Bhāvaprakāśa Pūrvakhaṇḍa 6.38–53 and 88–92

Then he named the components of medicine. The patient, the messenger, the physician, a long life span, money, a good attendant, and good medicine: these are the components of medicine according to the wise. (37) Then he named the characteristics of a patient. A patient is anyone who has a disease. It must be observed to what extent he should be treated, or indeed should not be treated, which is described subsequently. (38) Then he named the characteristics of one who should be treated. A patient who has a [good] constitution and a [good] appearance, who is resolute and has [good] eyesight, who is devoted to physicians and has conquered his senses should be treated by physicians. (39) Otherwise, a patient who is long-lived, resolute, wealthy, and has friends as well, who does as the physician says, and who is pious should be treated by physicians. (40) Then he named the characteristics of one who should not be treated. One who is violent, inconsiderate, cowardly, ungrateful, and inattentive, afflicted by sorrow, or not of a good family, one who is about to die, who lacks equipment, (41) who is an enemy, or who thinks himself a physician,[95] who is one who lacks piety, who is suspicious and not compliant with physicians: such a one is not to be treated by a physician. (42)

Then he spoke of the prohibition of medical treatment for those who should not be treated. By attending on such persons, a doctor would suffer many inconveniences. (43) Then he spoke of the characteristics of the messenger. One who comes to fetch the physician is called the messenger. And in which manner he is suitable is said here: (44) Messengers are of good birth, not deformed, and clever. They have clean clothes, and are pleasant, mounted on a horse or a bull, holding beautiful flowers and fruit. (45) They are of the same class and of good behavior, and they approach the physician in a place that has life[96] and at the right time on account of the comfort of the patient. (46) Now he spoke of the considerations concerning omens on the messenger's way. When the messenger goes to summon the physician for the patient, an omen that is of the nature of *soma*[97] is not auspicious, whereas one that is burning[98] conveys health. (47) Then he spoke of how the messenger and the patient should not approach the physician with empty hands. For instance, one would not approach a king, a physician, a preceptor, an astrologer, a god, or a friend with empty hands [but] with a fruit. This would yield a result. (48) Then he named the characteristics of a good physician. One who practices medicine is called a physician. In what manner he is good is described here. (49) A physician who has accurately studied the meaning of the teachings, has observed its practice and practiced himself, who is light-handed, clean, and strong, equipped with instruments and drugs, confident, sensible, and determined, who speaks kindly and who is honest and pious: such a physician is praised. (51) Then he spoke of the characteristics of the physician to be warded off. Badly clothed, rough, arrogant, vulgar, and come of his own accord: These five kinds of physician are not respected even when they are equal to Dhanvantari. (52) Then he spoke about the work of the physician. Accurate knowledge of disease and suppressing pain: That is what makes the physician's physicianhood. A physician is not the lord of life. (53) Then he reflected on life span. A physician should first examine the life span of an ill person with great care. If the life span is long, medical treatment will consequently be fruitful. (54)

Then he spoke of the necessity of money. Everyone needs money, including the patient, etc. Since there can be no remedy without money, money is a component of medicine. (88) Then he described the characteristics of the attendant. A friendly person who is not squeamish and strong, who is ready to care for the sick, follows the physician's orders, and is unwearying, is suitable as an attendant. (89) Then he spoke of the characteristics of the medicine. The substance with which the physician cures diseases is called medicine. He explained what is necessary so that it will remove diseases. (90) Then he gave a discourse on the harvesting of medicinal plants. A medicine that was grown in a

> suitable place and harvested on a suitable day and in small quantities, that has many good qualities and a (good) smell, color, and taste, that removes [excess] humors[99] and was abundant, that does not produce sickness and is administered after close examination and at [the right] time would produce good qualities. (91–92)

The *Bhāvaprakāśa* extends the list of four pillars of medicine into a list of seven components (*aṅga*, rather than *pāda*) by including messengers (*dūta*), a long life span (*dīrgham āyus*) and money (*dravya*). Their description is part of a chapter that discusses basic categorizations of disease and medicine. The added components of medicine—messengers, life span, and money—are given varying amounts of attention. Money, for example, is covered in a single sentence. Bhāvamiśra defines the need for money as a basic fact of human life. He argues that medical treatment cannot be done without medicines, which in turn cannot be attained without money. Money, then, is a prerequisite to the practice of medicine in a very real sense.

Defining the messenger as a component of medicine seems slightly more problematic and throws up some questions. Good messengers are defined by their outward appearance and behavior, but also by the time of their arrival, and even by the omens they encounter on their way to the physician. We will hear more about this later. The point is that, going by Bhāvamiśra's definition in 44–46, it is not their active participation in calling the physician to the patient's home that makes them an indispensable part of a medical setup. Instead, the messengers' contribution to medicine is to serve as—probably unwitting—omens of the course a patient's illness will take, allowing the physician to decide whether the patient's case is worth taking up or not. Messengers are therefore symptoms rather than participants. And thus, unless the messengers were aware of what they represented to the physician and therefore made sure to convey the right signals, their influence on medical treatment would have been indirect at best. The question that arises here concerns the use of messengers as a category: Why are messengers a component of medicine, but not what they stand for: omens or disease symptoms? Perhaps the subcategory of messengers is meant to represent the meta category of omens or symptoms, but this is not clear, since Bhāvamiśra does not elaborate.

The third additional component, a long life span, is only briefly discussed in one sentence. However, this is followed by a longer section on curable and incurable patients and the signs of impending death, which could be understood to pertain to the general topic of life span. The physician is advised that he should examine the patient's life span at the beginning, since treatment can only be successful if the patient has a long life span.

Both the knowledge of the life span and the signs represented by the messengers give the physician information about the likelihood of success in treatment, and this must necessarily be got prior to treatment. They could therefore be seen as preconditions to medical practice rather than as components of medical practice proper. In any case, neither the topic of messengers nor that of life span are innovations of Bhāvamiśra: we find corresponding descriptions in all of the older medical classics. Bhāvamiśra's novel contribution is to place them within the context of the components of medicine, adding them to the traditional four pillars. The case is slightly different with his added component of money, since money is a topic that most medical authors studiously avoid (see chapter 5). Bhāvamiśra not only speaks of money but places it at the center of medicine by including it as one of the components. This is a departure from the way the older texts handled (or rather, avoided) the subject and is thus Bhāvamiśra's innovation. In all other respects, the *Bhāvaprakāśa* does not differ from the views of the other authors, and in any case more or less copies the relevant passages from the *Suśrutasaṃhitā* and the *Carakasaṃhitā*.

The Physician, the Patient, and the Attendant

The Physician

The characteristics the medical authors attribute to the good physician within their four-pillar definitions can be broadly divided into two categories: The first are characteristics that pertain directly to the physician's medical knowledge and proficiency in practice, the "hard skills" of the medical profession. The Second are more general virtues, such as learnedness, as well as "soft skills": personality traits, social graces, personal habits, that is. The two categories can therefore be distinguished according to what makes someone a good person (or at least one that behaves well within a certain social context) and what qualifies him as a doctor. The boundaries between the two groups are somewhat fluid, at least in one direction, in that a good physician's characteristics must include both hard and soft skills. There is also some overlap in what could be deemed either a person's general positive characteristic or a more specifically medical one. For example, Suśruta's requirements that the physician be "light-handed, clean, and strong" could fit into either group. However, since all three attributes would be crucial for performing surgery, I am inclined to count them as professional qualifications. The word "knowledge" (*vidyā*) is a further ambiguous case: If it denotes medical knowledge, it belongs to the first group, if it means general knowledge, it belongs to the second. In his commentary on Ca.Sū.9.21, Cakrapāṇidatta posits "knowledge" firmly within the medical context, by glossing it with *vaidyakaśāstrajñāna*—"knowledge of medical science."[100] If we agree with Cakrapāṇidatta's interpretation, twenty out of twenty-four characteristics that Caraka gives belong to the first group, the physician's hard skills. Suśruta (about eight out of twelve) and Vāgbhaṭa (four out of four) show a similar bias toward medical proficiency in what they require of the good physician. Kaśyapa, on the other hand, emphasizes general good conduct and learnedness (only about eight hard skills out of twenty-two characteristics), while Bhāvamiśra mostly reiterates Suśruta's list, though he also adds "speaking kindly" to it. Only Caraka, however, demands soft skills that are directly connected to the physician's attitude to the patient: kindness to and compassion for the ill, affection for the remediable, and indifference or equanimity in regard to those who are healthy.[101]

All the medical authors require the physician to have studied and fully understood medical science on the one hand and to have extensive practical experience, both through observation and through performing treatment or surgery, on the other. The physician's command of both theory and practice is the sum total of his competence, on which the success of his treatments, that is, to cure or to prevent illnesses, rests. The conclusion that a physician must be in command of both theory and practice is reiterated in a number of other passages in the medical texts. Caraka states in Vi.8.86 that

> a physician, then, is one who heals, who is conversant with the meaning and the practical application of the aphoristic rules and by whom life is understood entirely and exactly. . . . These, then, are the qualities of the physician endowed with which a physician is capable of producing the normal state of the humors, namely thorough knowledge of the oral tradition, understanding of medical attendance, skill, cleanliness, manual dexterity, possession of medical equipment, possession of all senses, knowledge of the human constitution, and a knowledge of what ought to be done.

Suśruta in Sū.3.48–50 is not content with simply listing knowledge and experience as the basis of medical practice but argues more strongly that

> one who knows only the discipline's theory [*śāstra*] but is not completely skilled in medical practice becomes confused on meeting a patient, like a coward on reaching a battle. (48)
> However, one who is skilled in medical practice, but has set aside the discipline's theory out of boldness, is not well regarded by respectable people and meets with punishment by the king. (49)

Both are unskilled in and incapable of their practice with their half knowledge, like birds with only one wing. (50)[102]

Sheldon Pollock noted that the emphasis given to practice in medical literature (rather than giving "clear priority and absolute competence to shastric codification") is unusual and represents a minority stance in brahmanic literature, though a similarly dialectical formulation of the relation between theory and practice is also found in Kauṭilya's *Arthaśāstra.*[103]

If competence in both theory and practice is meant to ensure successful treatment, the keyword "success" should be the ultimate requirement of the physician. And indeed, Caraka asserts that "success shows the correct application of all measures, and success also shows the best physician who is endowed with all [good] qualities."[104] A close look into the prerequisites outlined by the medical authors above reveals that they may have had in mind, not only the needs of the ill but also the interests of the medical establishment they represented. We can infer this from (1) the postulation of a *śāstra*, a discipline with a circumscribed body of knowledge, which the physician is required to know, and (2) the assertion that there are formal ways in which this knowledge is to be received, that is, through "the teachings of a preceptor."[105] In other words, it is not enough that a person can cure or prevent illnesses: He must be able to do so from within a formal framework, using a certain set of knowledge and techniques. Point (2) deserves some discussion. As already briefly discussed, we find the reading *tīrthāttaśāstrārtha*, "who has received the meaning of the teachings from a preceptor" in the *Aṣṭāṅgahṛdayasaṃhitā* and the *Aṣṭāṅgasaṃgraha. Tīrtha* can also be translated as "in the right manner," but Aruṇadatta's commentary of the *Aṣṭāṅgahṛdayasaṃhitā* glosses it with *upādhyāya*, "teacher." Suśruta gives *tattvādhigataśāstrārtha*, "who has truly learnt the meaning of the teachings," instead. This is also the reading Suśruta's commentator Ḍalhaṇa favors, glossing it with *yathāvadadhītaśāstra*, "who has studied the teachings properly," and adding that this means having understood them properly. The *Bhāvaprakāśa* copies Suśruta's verse in Pūrv.6.50 and also reads *tattvādhigataśāstrārtha*. Trikamji, however, notes the alternative reading for Suśruta's verse *tīrthādhigataśāstrārtha*, "who has learnt the meaning of the teachings from a preceptor." Kaśyapa, again, lists "has a good teacher" (*sutīrtha*)[106] as a physician's requirement, while Caraka mentions "support" (*āśraya*), which Cakrapāṇidatta interprets as having the support of a teacher. There are other reasons that indicate that a physician's authority was derived at least partially from his connection with a particular teacher, and hence a particular school of thought: The classical treatises describe formal medical training at length. Suśruta, for example, gives a detailed description of the medical student's initiation in Sū.2.1–10, which includes instructions on the proper relationship between the student and the teacher.[107] Finally, Suśruta's words in Sū.4.8 leave no doubts about where he stands on this issue: "A physician who performs medical procedures, having heard the discipline transmitted through a teacher and having often repeated [it], is a [real] physician. The others are thieves." This conclusion points to a certain amount of competition on the medical market, in which claims of authority function as territorial stakes that fence off other competitors. Suśruta here allows only for two types of physician: the good, that is, the establishment physician, and the bad, that is, the nonestablishment practitioner.

Caraka, however, offers a third category:

> "Here are the three kinds of physicians:
> There are three kinds of physician in this world. One wears physician's disguise, another acquires sponsorship. But some do actually possess all the virtues of a true doctor.
> The impostors know nothing. They appropriate the title 'physician' by having doctor's trappings, medicines, and books, accompanied by posturing and pretence.
> Some, though unworthy, appropriate the title 'doctor' through the fiat of people who have achieved distinction, fame, and knowledge. These should be known as 'sponsored.'
> But there are persons who are truly accomplished in theory and practice who are knowledgeable and successful. They deliver comfort and are companions of life itself. The quality of the true doctor dwells in such as these."[108]

Here we have three categories: (1) the fraud; (2) the "sponsored" physician; and (3) the true physician. This categorization reasserts the notion of a competent physician as one "truly accomplished in theory and practice." However, the second category is perhaps the most interesting of the three. The concept of a "sponsored" physician who is in some undefined sense "unworthy" but nevertheless has some backing by authorities is somewhat ambiguous. To begin with, it raises the question who the "people who have achieved distinction, fame, and knowledge" are, that is, whether they are famous physicians or just eminent persons without a medical background. In either case, dubbing their protegés "unworthy" implies criticism of their judgment. If the distinguished persons are physicians, calling attention to their misjudgment could be understood as self-criticism from within the medical establishment. If they are not connected to medicine, this criticism could imply a bid for professional hegemony from medical men who would not accept the establishment of medical authority from without their group.

The word *atadvidha* in Ca.Sū.11.52 that Wujastyk renders as "unworthy" (interpreting *atadvidha* as "unlike" the knowledgeable) is probably a misreading for *atadvidya*, "nonexpert." Cakrapāṇidatta glosses it with *jñānahīna*, "without knowledge," or "deficient in knowledge," which confirms this reading. This gives persons belonging to this second category more or less the same standing as those in the first, the frauds. However, this second category could also be understood to represent practitioners who are not quite as good as true physicians, but who are still better than the frauds. Perhaps we may think of them as mediocre physicians. This distinction echoes remarks by Caraka in his passage on the four pillars of medicine, where he describes those practitioners of medicine who deserve the title *vaidya* and those who do not. The latter are "the ignorant physician" (*ājño bhiṣak*, Sū.9.15 and 16) and "the one who [merely] fancies himself a physician" (*bhiṣaṅmānin*, Sū.9.17). The "ignorant physician" could be the parallel of the "sponsored physician." While he may not deserve the title *vaidya*, he still is a *bhiṣak*, a physician, unlike the one who only thinks he is.[109] It is worth noting that, apart from in this context, we do not find another instance of this distinction between *vaidya* and *bhiṣak*; these titles generally seem interchangeable.

To summarize, we have encountered the following five categories so far:

1. The good physician who deserves the title *vaidya*
2. The "sponsored" physician
3. The ignorant physician
4. The one who merely believes himself a physician
5. The fraud/quack

The last three of these probably describe more or less the same thing, while the second is a somewhat uncertain case. However, it leans more toward the fraud than toward the good physician, particularly if we go with Cakrapāṇidatta's interpretation of *atadvidha* as "without knowledge." Thus, in the end, we are left with the polar opposites of good and bad physicians.

Caraka certainly leaves behind the notion of mediocrity, not-quite-good-enough, or indeed any other subtle differentiation when he offers the contrasting categories of "savers of life and destroyers of disease" and "savers of disease and destroyers of life" in Sū.29.5.[110] We have encountered the "saver of life" before, in Ca.Sū.9.18, where he is characterized as "one who is engaged in the set of four: the discipline, comprehension of its meaning, its application, and the observation of medical practice." In Ca.Sū.29, we learn more about this life-saving physician. Caraka begins with this short definition: "The wise person who has knowledge of these,[111] the sense organs, the intellect [*vijñāna*], the cause of consciousness, and disease is truly called a 'saver of life.' "[112] This summary is notably different from the one of Ca.Sū.9.18, in that it does not lay out the tools of the trade, as it were, but concerns knowledge of a human's cognitive faculties. The mention of the sense organs and of the intellect may be a reference to Caraka's list of threes in Sū.11, in which the "inappropriate conjunction of objects and senses, [and] the violation of good judgment"[113] (*prajñāparādha*) are declared two of three causes of disease. Following on from this, Caraka gives a list of "saver-of-life essentials" that refer to the contents of the Sūtrasthāna chapter by chapter. This list begins with some familiar attributes of the physician's trade skills:

> There are those who are well-born and accomplished in their discipline, who have observed practice and are skilled and clean, whose hands are trained and whose self is controlled, who have all equipment and who have their wits about them, who know about natural states and about procedures: these are known as savers of life and destroyers of disease.[114]

Two of these attributes are new to our good physician's checklist: The requirement that a physician be well-born (*kūlina*) does not occur in the four-pillar definitions.[115] It is, however, found in a passage on the selection of a medical student in the *Suśrutasaṃhitā*.[116] Caraka's parallel passage in Vi.8.8 asks more specifically for the student to come from a family of physicians.[117] The second characteristic that stands out in the above quote is that the savers of life should be self-controlled (*jitātman*). I have not found this elsewhere in the medical classics as a requirement of the physician. Then, Caraka's list begins in earnest, as the minutiae of what a physician should know are detailed in the rest of Sū.29.7. As it turns out, Caraka would have a physician know the contents of the Sūtrasthāna: the items in the list match each of its chapters one by one, with some exceptions.[118] Only at the end of the seventh sentence do we arrive back at more general merits:

> [Those] who are competent in mindfulness, understanding, the discipline, and knowledge of [its] application, with good conduct, always keeping their word, entertaining friendly thoughts toward all beings as if they were mother, father, brother, or relative: such [physicians], Agniveśa, are savers of life and destroyers of diseases.

Two of the above characteristics, namely "good conduct" and "entertaining friendly thoughts toward all beings," and so on, represent the divide between etiquette, that is, the prescribed limits of appropriate social behavior within a set situation, and ethics: the moral judgment of behavior according to a particular set of values. The two are intertwined, since prescriptions of conduct may have moral underpinnings.

As noted, Caraka's good physician, the "saver of life" of Sū.29, is contrasted with "the saver of disease" and "destroyer of life," the quack. The quack is the good physician's antithesis, his opposite in behavior, knowledge, skill, and ethics. We have met him in the previous chapters: Caraka describes him in his four-pillar definition as one who makes curable illnesses worse, and likens him to a blind person groping around helplessly or a boat controlled by the wind.[119] This quack is misguided in thinking that he can practice medicine: By chance he had success once, due to the fixed life span of the patient. Believing himself a physician, he then wreaks havoc on the rest of his patients, even to the point of killing them. He is ignorant, and perhaps vain, and therefore completely misjudges his abilities. The word used by Caraka in Sū.9.17, *bhiṣaṅmānin*, "one who believes himself a physician," implies that his misjudgment is genuine, and that while such a person may do great damage to his hapless patients, he does so without evil intent. Such a quack may be as much a danger to himself as to the patient. Suśruta, for example, describes a quack surgeon who cuts himself when attempting surgery.[120]

Interestingly, it seems that the medical authors would have the patient himself bear the responsibility for choosing a good physician. Caraka notes that "it is better to burn oneself than be administered medicine by one who is ignorant."[121] And Suśruta cautions that "a prudent person who wishes to live a long life" ought to avoid bad physicians, "like an angry poisonous snake."[122] To be able to avoid quacks, patients would have to be capable of judging for themselves whether a physician is ignorant or knowledgeable. This would require a high level of discernment from them, similar to the competence patients are meant to display when describing their illnesses.[123] Conversely, an incompetent patient who falls prey to a quack is implicitly criticized: The fault is at least partly his, since he has made an error of judgment. As Siegel (1987, 176) puts it, "it is our blindness that allows us to be hoodwinked by the crooked quack, the venal *vaidya*—the vice is his, but the folly is ours." But is this truly so?

When Caraka lays out the three kinds of physician in Ca.Sū.11.50–53, he names two kinds of physician that do not meet the standards of the true physician: One who "wears physician's disguise" and another who "acquires sponsorship." The "sponsored" physicians seem to fit the quack described above, with one difference: It is not only their own misjudgment that lets them fancy themselves physicians but also that of the authorities who support them.[124] Those who disguise themselves as physicians, on the other hand, are characterized as actively fraudulent. They "appropriate the title 'physician' by having doctor's trappings, medicines, and books, accompanied by posturing and pretence."[125] Siegel (1987, 168) also argues that "there is intimidating power in noncomprehended language. The doctor's rhetoric is an armor that safeguards status and conceals a lack of the very knowledge that it is supposed to express." Keeping in mind that neither support by authorities nor outward appearances could be trusted, the patient's difficulty in discerning correctly whether a physician was the real thing or not can hardly be judged a folly. The odds are against the patient. There are, however, some clues that separate the quack's behavior from that of a true physician. Caraka describes these in Sū.29.8–9:[126]

> Then there are their opposites, the savers of diseases and destroyers of life, those who disguise themselves as physicians, thorns to mankind, counterfeits without morals who roam countries because of their rulers' carelessness. (8)
>
> 'Attired in doctors' outfits, they wander the streets looking for work. As soon as they hear that someone is ill, they descend on him and in his hearing speak loudly of their medical expertise. If a doctor is already in attendance on him, they constantly harp on that doctor's failings. They try to ingratiate themselves with the patient's friends with jokes, confidences, and flattery. They put it about that they won't want much money.... [having found a case, they constantly observe, wishing to conceal their ignorance with (feigned) skill,][127] but when they fail to avert the illness they point out that it was the patient himself who lacked equipment, helpers, and the right attitude.[128]
>
> Having noticed that his (i.e., the patient's) end has come near, they go to some other place under some pretext. When they meet ordinary people, they describe their own skill like fools. Like those deficient in self-command, they criticize the composure of those who are in self-command. When they see learned persons, they avoid them the way travelers avoid a dangerous forest from afar. When they have taken to some part of an aphoristic rule, they constantly quote it whether relevant or not. They do not wish to question, nor to be questioned, and shrink from questions as from death. And no one is known as their teacher, pupil, costudent, or disputant.

This passage reads as satire, especially the ironic titles of "savers of disease" and "destroyers of health" that Caraka uses for the frauds. According to this section, it is mostly their behavior (i.e., not their treatments) that gives them away as charlatans:

1. They actively seek out patients without having been called.
2. They act in a too familiar manner with the patient's friends and family.
3. They brag about their own abilities.
4. They denigrate the abilities of other physicians but avoid direct confrontation.
5. They shirk from any encounter with other physicians that would allow for a direct comparison of their abilities, or for their methods to be questioned.
6. Nothing is known of their medical provenance.
7. They quote inappropriately from medical or other authoritative works.
8. They blame the patient if their treatment fails, saying that he lacked equipment, helpers, and the right attitude.
9. They leave the patient under some pretext if they realize that he is about to die.

Of these, the first six are useful pointers for the patient and should set off the warning bells. Such behavior stands in complete contrast to the good physician's standard etiquette,[129] and can be easily recognized even by those who would not be able to discern real from faked knowledge. Number 7 is a borderline case: One cannot expect the general populace to be familiar with learned treatises. However, it may just be a matter of common sense to know when someone is quoting texts inappropriately. The last two characteristics only apply in hindsight once the damage has been done. These are peculiar points, since they describe attitudes that come close to what is described elsewhere as acceptable standards of good medical practice. After all, according to four-pillar definitions, a good patient should be equipped with what is necessary for treatment, and he should follow the physician's orders, and so on. As we have seen, the question whether a patient must have the necessary equipment is debated by the medical authors in terms of whether or not a physician should take up treatment for a patient who lacks adequate equipment. Theoretically, this means the lack of equipment should no longer be an issue once a physician has decided to give treatment. However, one can easily imagine this to have been an ongoing concern. Noncompliance of patients—if this is what we understand "lacks the right attitude" stands for—is a genuine problem in medical care, and could indeed lead to the failure of treatment. And, as I discuss later, the physician is held to give up patients who are about to die. Presumably, a good physician would not leave the patient under some pretext, though how exactly he would proceed is not explained in the treatises. This situation offers a dilemma to the good physician, since he is not meant to treat someone who is about to die, but he is also not supposed to tell either the patient or the patient's family or friends of the patient's imminent death if he judges that this will upset them. What other course of action remains open in such a case than to leave the patient under some pretext? This goes to show how the line between the actions of a good physician and those of a quack may become blurred. A real difference would be one of intent, but the medical authors do not offer a discussion of that.

Two more points stand out in Caraka's passage. One is the idea that it is somehow the ruler's fault if quacks practice medicine within his state. Suśruta suggests the same in Sū.3.52, where he states that the bad physician kills people through the fault of the king. Scharfe (2002, 261) calls attention to the fact that neither the medical texts nor other sources give evidence of examinations administered or supervised by the state, and concludes that "the king's guilt in such cases was no different from his guilt if people in his state acted unlawfully—or his merit if they followed a moral path. His only way of actively rooting out bad medicine lay in punishing bad physicians for injuries or death due to malpractice."

This links up with the other point worth noting in Ca.Sū.29.8: Caraka's use of the epithet "thorns" (*kaṇṭaka*) to describe quacks. This usage also occurs in book 4 of Kauṭilya's *Arthaśāstra*, where physicians are listed among artisans as potential thorns to society, that is, criminals. The relevant clause of the *Arthaśāstra* (4.1.56) refers specifically to offenses committed by physicians during their work. The main offense is not to notify the authorities about dangerous procedures prior to undertaking them, and punishments are meted out according to the results of treatment: death of the patient through no fault of the physician, death of the patient due to medical error, or deformity of the patient due to malpractice. This tells us a number of things: First, that a physician who notifies the authorities of a dangerous procedure is working within the established system. Second, that the notification serves as insurance against being punished for unsuccessful treatment. Accordingly, it seems that unsuccessful treatment was acceptable as long as the authorities were informed of this possible outcome beforehand, and even medical error would not constitute an offense per se. Interpreted cynically, this means that a physician whose treatments failed was not a quack, as long as he operated within the system.

Bhāvamiśra offers another take on the subject of quacks. In his definition of the components of medicine, he sketches a portrait of physicians one should avoid: "Badly clothed, rough, arrogant, vulgar, and come of his own accord: These five kinds of physician are not respected even when they are equal to Dhanvantari."[130] This definition is extraordinary in that Bhāvamiśra seems to weigh the physician's appearance and behavior against his knowledge and skill, and judges the former characteristics to be of greater importance than the latter. To be a brilliant doctor—equal to the physician of the gods!—is not enough to gain respect and acceptance from the public. A physician also needs to conform to a certain standards of behavior and to take care of his appearance. This makes sense if we remember that the patient really only had the physician's behavior to go by when trying to decide whether he was respectable or a quack. Being badly clothed, for instance, points to a disregard for social custom that might entail other inappropriate behavior. It may also indicate poverty (as opposed to poor taste in clothing), and this in itself would have been a sign of failure in a physician. Being rough, arrogant, or vulgar are all characteristics that contrast with the behavior of a genteel and learned person, and calling at a patient's house without having been summoned is the ultimate faux pas that a respectable and established physician would never commit.[131] The question is, however, why he wouldn't. Basham claims that the physician was not forbidden to advertise his skill, and refers to the Vinaya piṭaka (*Mahāvagga* 8.1.8–13), which describes how Jīvaka, the great physician of Buddhist legend, comes to Sāketa and calls out on the streets: "Who is ill here? Whom shall I cure?"[132] This may imply an answer being called out: "I am ill. Come and treat me!" (or more likely: "My master is ill, come and treat him!") and this could perhaps be considered a summoning of the physician. However, Jīvaka, the physician in this scenario, is part of a *śramana* system (i.e., of wandering ascetics) that functions outside the settled community, both in terms of physical location and of values and beliefs. He comes to a town as an outsider and, from the perspective of the (brahmanic) establishment, as a disturbance to their order of life. After all, a cure from a Buddhist healer may effect the conversion of the patient. According to Zysk (2000, 4), the origins of medical practice as laid out in the medical classics go back to heterodox śramanic traditions. He states that "heterodox ascetic intellectuals accumulated, systematized, and transmitted a body of medical lore that was later assimilated and processed by Brāhmaṇs to fit into an orthodox Weltanschauung." The notion, then, that a physician should only come when he is called may in the end go back to a rivalry between settled physicians who belonged to the brahmanic establishment and wandering healers, and it may thus be an example of established physicians breaking with the unorthodox past of the medical trade.

However, we do not actually gain a very clear picture from the medical treatises of whether their physician is envisioned as a settled and established citizen of a town or county or as an itinerant practitioner. There are pointers to either possibility: There is mention of roaming about practicing medicine after medical studies have been completed (in the teacher's speech to the medical student in Ca.Vi.8.13), implying at least a phase of wandering around offering medical services. Conversely, the notion that it is bad conduct to come when not summoned presupposes that a physician had a place from which he could be summoned: a fixed abode, or at least a place in which he could be routinely found.

If a physician did live as a member of a community, he would have been a known quantity to the other inhabitants. His lifestyle, including his religious and cultural leanings, would have been under scrutiny, and his successes and failures in medicine would have been widely known. There is some epigraphical evidence that physicians in later years at least had fixed appointments (being affiliated with a temple, for example).[133]

However, even established physicians were not exempt from criticism, as we know from other sources. Siegel (1985, 1987) has shown that satirical medieval Indian literature provides a particularly rich mine of information on how physicians were perceived.[134] In this genre, there is no such thing as a good physician—any physician is a quack by default, marked not only by incompetence but also by hypocrisy, prurience, cowardice, and greed. Siegel (1987, 177) gives a striking rendition of some verses in Sūrya's *Sūktiratnahāra* (136.6) that refer to the physician's cowardice and greed:

> He can't extend the life you've led
> Though for that he'll charge his fees:
> His skill's in running from the dead
> And in performing moneyectomies!

Money and medicine is a recurring theme in medical satire. The patient pays doubly: with his money and with his health, or even his life. Of course, the satirized physician always does damage to the patient, and his fees are thus inherently unfair. However, the fact that a physician's fees so often form the central topic of satire may point to a more general unease about the connection between a patient's illness and a physician's income. The classical medical authors display a certain guardedness on the topic of a physician's livelihood and never mention fees outright. In Ca.Sū.29.9, a hypocritical attitude toward money is one of the characteristics of a quack: "They put it about that they won't want much money." This implies that money is, in fact, foremost on the quack's mind. It also suggests that patients expected to pay for a doctor's services, that there were no fixed rates, and that these fees may have been a point of contention. I discuss this further in chapter 5.

To conclude, the *Carakasaṃhitā* is our main source on quacks in the Sanskrit medical classics, though short comments from the *Suśrutasaṃhitā* and the *Bhāvaprakāśa* complete the picture Caraka sketches. Caraka describes two types of quacks: one is a deluded person who wrongly, though perhaps innocently, believes himself to be a physician. The other is someone who knows full well that he lacks knowledge and skill yet viciously persists in practicing medicine. The result in either case is the same: damage to the patient whose illness is not only not cured but in some cases even exacerbated. This is, however, seen as the patient's own fault, since he should have had the good sense to establish whether his doctor was a good physician or a fraud in the first place. The physician's behavior provides the patient with the necessary information to make this decision. Bad behavior, such as bragging, speaking badly of others, being inappropriately familiar or arrogant signify that a person cannot be trusted. His physical appearance, particularly his dress, gives further clues. Finally, if a physician comes unbidden, a patient can be certain that he is dealing with a quack. Satirical literature adds greed to the bad physician's failings and highlights the uneasy relationship between money and medicine.

By contrast, the good physician's behavior is characterized by his knowledge and skill, and his adherence to etiquette and the ethics that underlie it. His main mark of identification lies in his success as a physician: the number of cures connected with his treatments. The results of his success are wealth and a good reputation, and these in turn serve to further inform the patient about his abilities.

The Patient

The patient is omnipresent in the medical classics as a carrier of disease and its symptoms. He is the subject of the physician's study and scrutiny and the recipient of the physician's diagnosis and administrations. Yet we learn surprisingly little about him, and even less about the interaction between him and the physician. The medical treatises offer no case histories that would flesh out the patient's image.[135] We learn more about persons that a physician should not accept as patients than about those that he should. And in either case, it is how the choice of patient reflects on the physician that is discussed by the medical authors. Therefore, some of the sections that mention the patient are dealt with in the section on the physician rather than here.

In Caraka's, Suśruta's, and Vāgbhaṭa's four-pillar definitions, the patient—the *ātura* (suffering, diseased), *vyādhyupasṛṣṭa* (afflicted by illness), *vyādhita* (ill), or *rogin* (sick)—is quickly described. Caraka's patient is mindful, obedient, fearless, and gives information on his disease. Suśruta's list is a bit more extensive. His patient is long-lived, resolute, curable, wealthy, prudent, pious, and attentive to what the doctor says. Vāgbhaṭa picks "wealthy, obedient to the physician, providing information, and resolute" from Caraka's and Suśruta's characteristics. Kaśyapa has similar things to say about the patient and gives more particulars. According to him, the perfect patient has a curable disease. He[136] is of a stable nature, strength, mind, body, sense-organs, will, and vital power. He gives exact information on his disease, its causes, early symptoms, its development, whether he has pain, whether there were any complications, and which medication is suitable or unsuitable for him. He (or in this case more likely she) should have faith in the wet-nurse. Pious, well-behaved, obedient, and self-controlled, the patient should give respect to the gods, the twice-born, teachers, physicians, medicines, and friends. Kaśyapa's patient in fact seems hardly in need of a doctor at all, since apart from whatever ailment needs attending to, he is basically very healthy and knows exactly what his disease is and where it came from. This image of a well-informed patient is particularly surprising given that Kaśyapa's treatise is on *kaumārabhṛtya*, the care of young children (and pregnant or lying–in women, as well as wet-nurses).

Kaśyapa's perfect patient uses his knowledge of his disease by giving the physician full and clear information on his condition. Caraka briefly touches on this in his summary of the patient's qualities in Sū.9.9 with the phrase "jñāpakatvaṃ ca rogāṇām," (providing information on illnesses); Vāgbhaṭa abbreviates Caraka's phrase to *jñāpakaḥ*, "a provider of information." Kaśyapa's depiction of this process is more fully developed, as he demands of the patient "exact communication of causes, early symptoms, pain, complications, development, and suitable and nonsuitable medication." This is as close as any of the medical authors gets to describing active patient participation in the medical process. Kaśyapa may owe the particular requirement of patient participation to Buddhist sources: We find a parallel description to Kaśyapa's in Buddhist literature. The *Mahāvagga* states the following about good patients:

> The qualities of a patient easy to nurse are as follows: he does what is beneficial; he knows moderation in what is beneficial; he takes his medicine; *he makes clear the affliction, as it arises, to the nurse and wishes him well, saying "it is progressing" as it progresses, "it is regressing" as it*

> *regresses, and "it is stable" as it stabilizes*; and he endures the arising of bodily sensations that are painful, acute, sharp, severe, disagreeable, unpleasant, and destructive.[137]

The information the patient is meant to provide corresponds to the information a physician should elicit from the patient described in the *Suśrutasaṃhitā* (Sū.10.4–5). In a passage describing the physician's professional conduct, Suśruta explains how the physician should go about diagnosis: "Then, having taken a seat, he should have a good look at the patient, feel him, and question him."[138] Suśruta specifies that a physician should elicit information about "place, time, birth station [i.e., class background], things which are compatible, the onset of the illness, the buildup of pain, the strength, the digestion, the production or otherwise of wind, urine, and feces, about the dominant condition at a particular moment, and so forth."[139] Suśruta does not mention providing information as a requirement of the patient.

Finally, Kaśyapa is the only author to raise the possibility that the patient may be the most important of the four pillars, "since it is for his sake that the other three pillars are desired to be full of merit."[140] This notion is, however, hastily discarded in the next verse, where Prajāpati as the ultimate voice of authority posits that the physician is the most important of the four.

Obedience to the physician is at the core of the patient–physician relationship. Following the physician's orders is important for the success of therapy, which in turn reflects on the physician's competence. The medical authors seem to envisage a fairly passive patient who simply receives the physician's (or the attendants') ministrations and advice. He is required to take up a certain regime for the duration of treatment (though adhering to the tenets of *svasthavṛtta*, healthy lifestyle, is recommended to all at all times), but therapy generally seems to consist of things done *to* him rather than *by* him. Patient participation—apart from in the shape of the patient giving the physician information on his condition—does not figure as a desirable element of therapeutic interaction. Patient resistance, on the other hand, is clearly categorized as unacceptable: A patient who will not follow the physician's orders may even be abandoned by the physician. Caraka, however, records one instance of patient resistance in which the physician may take resort to another solution: In Ca.Cik.8.149–157, he describes how a physician may lie to a patient vis-à-vis the use of certain meats in a medicinal diet. I will discuss this passage in greater detail in chapter 6, but the passage is also of interest here as it records the patient's voice of dissent, albeit obliquely. Caraka explains why the physician may have to lie about the meats he wishes to administer to the patient:

> He should employ deception about those meats that aren't liked because they are unusual, because that way they can be eaten easily. Knowing what it was, feeling disgusted, the patient would not even eat, or would cause what was eaten to come up again. Therefore, he should let such meats be administered after they have been disguised.

We hear the patient's voice like that of a spoilt child here: "Yuk! I won't eat that!" And indeed, the paternalistic assumption that underlies this scenario—namely that the physician knows better than the patient what is good for him—places the physician in the role of parent and the patient in the role of child, and a petulant one at that. The passage very much exemplifies the top-down relationship between physician and patient. It conjures up the image of a superior physician who decides and acts according to his own discretion, and of a patient who is trusting and ready to be guided (he lets himself be deceived, after all) but at the same time potentially mutinous. Caraka clearly does not understand dissent and noncompliance or even informed consent as the patient's prerogative. On the contrary, the criticizing patient is viewed as a danger to himself, which justifies the physicians tricking him into compliance.

Caraka gives us some insight into the patient demographic in Siddhisthāna 11.28–30:

> Then Agniveśa asked about persons who are always ill and about their welfare, and the teacher replied: "Learned brahmins, the king's servants, and likewise courtesans, together with tradesmen are always ill. The twice-born with his studies of the Veda, vows, and daily rituals etc. neglects his body's welfare; the king's servant because of acting according to the king's wishes or fulfilling others' wishes, because of having much on his mind or out of fear. The courtesan who caters to men's wishes, is completely devoted to service, and is intent on her complexion and ornaments [neglects her health, as does] the tradesman, because of always sitting, overattachment to selling and buying etc., and greed etc. They always suppress their natural urges, do not eat meals on time, excrete and move around at wrong times.[141] They, and also others are always ill."[142]

Note that these potential patients are likely to be wealthy persons (possibly with the exception of the wider category of the twice-born, i.e., learned brahmins). The question of a patient's wealth is raised several times by the medical authors. Suśruta and Vāgbhaṭa list wealth as one of the patient's characteristics in their four-pillar definitions. Vāgbhaṭa also notes elsewhere that health shows in a patient who "has considerable amounts of money, who has good qualities, devotion to physicians and the twice-born, and a regard for medicine."[143]

Yet that an ideal patient should be wealthy does not necessarily translate into the maxim that a physician should only treat one from whom he can expect remuneration. For example, Suśruta stipulates that physicians should provide free treatment for some select persons:

> The twice-born, teachers, the poor, friends, mendicants, one's dependents, respectable persons, orphans, and those approaching [for help] should be treated with one's own medicine like one's own relatives: that is good.... Thus knowledge shines and one attains friends, fame, religious merit, wealth, and pleasure.[144]

In another place, Suśruta lists the poor among those who are extremely difficult to treat.[145] His commentator Ḍalhaṇa explains that this is due to their not being able to afford medicines.[146] Caraka goes one step further in saying that poor persons should not be treated at all.[147] Cakrapāṇidatta explains that a poor person would not have the necessary equipment for treatment, which would mean that therapy could not succeed.[148] The reason for not treating a poor person would therefore not be that such a patient could not generate income for the physician but that a poor person would not have the means to see treatment through.

The question of the pecuniary relationship between patient and physician is only briefly discussed in the medical classics. Caraka notes that "any clever person wishing to have a long life should not wish evil upon or speak or act badly toward a master of life. A person who has been treated, but does not recompense the physician, still owes him, whether agreed to or not."[149] The verb I have translated as "recompense," *upa-kṛ*, does not necessarily imply monetary rewards. It could mean any act performed to assist or benefit the physician in some way. I will return to this topic in chapter 5.

From the foregoing quotations, it appears that the patient demographic is constituted of children, pregnant and lying-in women, wet-nurses, learned brahmins, the king's servants, courtesans, tradesmen, teachers, the poor (unless we go with Caraka's verdict that they should not be treated), friends, mendicants, the physician's dependents, respectable persons, orphans, and those approaching the physician for help. To this, we can add Zimmermann's patient par excellence, the king.[150] Incidentally, nearly all of these are named by Suśruta as difficult to treat.[151] The *Aṣṭāṅgasaṃgraha* gives a little information about the king as a patient, stating that he and his retinue are "vulnerable to diseases on account of their way of living."[152] Acting recklessly and resorting to unwholesome pleasures, they are at the same time unable to put up with pain.[153] As.Sū.8.96–110 records a code of conduct for the king's physician, which warns the physician to be very careful indeed around the powerful and impatient king, avoiding any conflict with him and generally cosseting him while attracting as little attention to his own person as possible. This gives the impression that it must have been a very difficult and perhaps even dangerous post, requiring tact and discretion, and even a good amount of sycophancy. Such a king would certainly not have been an easy patient. Suśruta, however, explains that the king deserves special attention and respect due to his position. He also ascribes to the king the qualities of forbearance and steadfastness, qualities that would in fact make the king a good patient:

> There is merely a likeness in form between men and kings. [The king's] authority, liberality, forbearance, steadfastness and valor [make him] superhuman. Hence, the wise physician, desiring [his own] welfare, should constantly mind the king like a god, with pleasant speech, mind, and actions.[154]

While the above list probably covers much of the population, the medical authors also have lists of undesirables whom physicians are cautioned not to treat. For example, Suśruta advises in Sū.2.8 that "hunters, bird-catchers, the degraded, and evildoers should not be treated." Caraka's blacklist in Vi.3.45 is longer:

> One who does not oppose slander, who is poor, who does not have servants, who believes himself a physician, who is violent and discontented, who indulges in extremely unrighteous acts, whose strength, flesh, and blood are too depleted, who is afflicted with an incurable disease, and who shows the signs of impending death: by attending upon such a patient, a physician gets saddled with a bad reputation. On this, there is this verse: "If actions might have bad consequences in the present or in the future, they should not be done. That is the opinion of wise men."

Caraka complements his initial list with another one in Si.2.4–6:

> One who is violent, inconsiderate, cowardly, ungrateful, and inattentive, an enemy of respectable persons, kings, and doctors, or despised by them, someone afflicted by sorrow, who acts at random and who is about to die, who lacks equipment, who is an enemy or a quack, who is one who lacks faith, who is suspicious and not compliant to physicians:

> such a one is not to be treated by a physician. By attending on such persons, a doctor would suffer many inconveniences.

There are further comparable lists in Ca.Vi.8.13 (see p. xxx) and in Bhāv.Pūrv.6.41–42 (see p. xx). Ah.Sū.1.34–35ab and As.Sū.2.18-19 repeat much of Caraka's list in Si.2.4–6, and supplement it with persons who are "very old."[155]

Caraka gives a reason why these persons should not be treated: Treating them would give the physician a bad reputation, and he would suffer "inconveniences" or "bad consequences" (*doṣa*) of some sort. The nature of these inconveniences or bad consequences may depend on what characterizes the listed persons as undesirables. Treating those who stand in conflict with authorities—the king, respectable persons, other physicians—might mean angering or falling out of favor with the said authorities. The motive for staying away from such patients would therefore be political and/or social. Treating someone who "is violent, inconsiderate, cowardly, [and] ungrateful" would be difficult in itself. Such a person would certainly be unpleasant to treat. A physician also might not like to associate with someone of lowly behavior, since this could reflect badly on himself and thus have social implications. The reason not to treat such a patient could also be moral, in that a bad person might be deemed undeserving of medical attention. In his commentary on Ca.Si.2.4–6, Cakrapāṇidatta explains that it would be unrighteous to treat such persons, but also that medicines would not work on them:

> In the case of violent persons, the efficacy [*pravṛtti*] of the medicine is suppressed because it is impotent, and where ingrates are concerned, the medicine doesn't cure because of the power of unrighteousness. In fact, by helping the unrighteous, unrighteousness arises. Thus, restraint is the rule.[156]

Those who are inattentive, are suspicious, fancy themselves physicians, and are not compliant to the physician, as well as those who are afflicted by sorrow or who act at random, may be grouped into another category. The common denominator here is noncompliance, the ultimate result of which is that effective treatment becomes impossible.[157] Lastly, physicians are cautioned not to treat those who are very old and those who are about to die. The patient who is about to die is given much attention by the medical authors, and we will have a closer look at this subject later.

As regards the other undesirables, some of them are also mentioned in other contexts as persons anyone should avoid. Suśruta, for example, notes in his account of good conduct (*sadvṛtta*) in Cik.24.90 that

> one should not say what is hated by the king, harsh, slanderous, or untrue, and one should not speak against gods, brahmins, or forefathers. Nor should one associate with persons hated by the king, [or] those who are mad, fallen, lowly, or inferior.

Caraka gives a similar list as part of his code of good conduct in Sū.8.19, where he admonishes that one should not keep company with unrighteous persons, with those who are hated by the king, with those who are mad, fallen, lowly, or corrupted, and finally, with abortionists.[158]

The reward for staying away from such persons (and for keeping to the other rules of good conduct) is to acquire religious merit, wealth, and pleasure and to earn the friendship of all living beings.[159] This is very similar to what Suśruta says about offering medical treatment to the right persons (i.e., the twice-born, teachers, the poor, friends, etc.) in Sū.2.8, where he concludes: "Thus knowledge shines and one attains friends, fame, religious merit, wealth, and pleasure." The relationship between a physician and his patients therefore parallels the relationships between persons in society in general. What is considered good for the physician is also good for any member of the public.

To summarize and conclude, the medical authors' image of the patient is very much derived from the perspective of the physician's needs. Most of the patient's good characteristics—wealth, curability, obedience to the physician, and fearlessness—pertain to the physician's convenience: A good patient is one who makes the physician's job easy and worthwhile.

A patient's participation in his treatment is limited to aiding the physician through giving accurate information on his condition. In this, he is competent. He may not, however, entertain ideas of his own about how to treat himself, nor may he refuse the physician's advice or administrations. Obedience to the physician and compliance with his orders are the patient's greatest virtues. Conversely, thinking himself a physician and noncompliance make him someone a physician would reject.

The patient demographic seems to represent a good portion of the population. It comprises a diverse range of people, such as the poor and courtesans, brahmins and the nobility. All of these were probably considered respectable society by the medical authors. In the case of poor people, we find one of the rare instances of dissension among the authors' views: Caraka suggests outright that poor people should not be treated. His commentator Cakrapāṇidatta attempts to soften this dictum by explaining that a poor person could not afford to see treatment through, which would make medical intervention useless. However, Suśruta takes the opposite stance, while fully acknowledging that medical treatment of poor persons is difficult. He judges that a physician should treat poor people as if they were family, which I take to mean "for free."

Otherwise, the medical authors concur in their lists of which patients should be rejected. Analyzing these, it seems safe to suggest that the persons a physician should not treat divide into two main categories: (1) social outcasts that anyone concerned with their reputation would wish to avoid, and (2) persons whose treatment would fail. The latter, though respectable members of society, must be avoided by the physician, since he may be held responsible for their continued illness or death.

Finally, it must be noted that while the medical treatises give us some idea of who the patients were and how they interacted with the physician, the image they project is barely fleshed out. The patient as a person remains strangely absent, perhaps due to the lack of case histories. Nearly everything we learn about the patient relates to the physician, so that, in the end, we learn more about the latter than about the patient.

The Attendant and Other Helpers

In the context of the four pillars, Caraka, Suśruta, and Vāgbhaṭa are brief in what they say about the perfect attendant. According to Caraka, he knows how to attend, [and] is skillful, clean, and full of affection.[160] Suśruta would have him friendly, accepting, and strong, ready to care for the sick, obedient to the physician, and unwearying, and Vāgbhaṭa's attendant is affectionate, clean, able, and intelligent.[161] However, Kaśyapa envisages a rather more distinguished attendant who, apart from being healthy, strong, clean, and swift, is also able to prepare medicinal decoctions and excels in his knowledge of medical practice, his skill, and his experience in all treatments. This perfect attendant is devoted to his master, is unsqueamish, and comes from a good family. He is straightforward, self-controlled, and patient, having conquered anger and other vices.[162] Thus, Kaśyapa's attendant hardly seems a step down from the physician. Indeed, his checklist of characteristics is strikingly similar to what Suśruta gives on the physician in Kalp.1.8–11:

> [The king] should employ in his kitchens a doctor who is respected by his peers and who, in addition to a good stock of medicines, is endowed with the following virtues: Someone well-bred, orthodox, sympathetic, [well-paid,] and always at the ready. A person who is neither greedy, nor false, but devoted, appreciative, and nice-looking, and in whom there is no anger, coarseness, jealousy, fraudulence, or idleness. He should be in control of his senses, have patience, be clean and full

> of kindness and good manners. Someone intelligent, energetic, loyal, and well-intentioned. Someone sharp, profound, penetrating, deft, and dynamic.[163]

Yet Kaśyapa concurs with the other authors in the judgment that an attendant is subsidiary to the physician. I have already briefly raised the question of the medical attendant's status within society, asking who would have been ready to undertake this sullying work and be acceptable to patients at the same time. Suśruta's note that an attendant should be not squeamish and ready to care for the sick indicates that this may have been a problem. Kaśyapa mentions that an attendant should not have lowly family connections (*akṣudraputratva*) but does not discuss the implications of the nature of the work for the attendant's status. Unfortunately, we learn no more about this question from the medical classics. However, other sources do provide some insight into this topic. For example, the problem of the nurse–patient relationship is tackled head-on in Buddhist literature. Zysk makes note of a passage in the *Mahāvagga* in which the Buddha lectures the monks about their responsibilities toward each other in the case of illness: "You, O *bhikkhus*, have neither a mother nor a father who could nurse you. If, O *bhikkhus*, you do not nurse one another, who, then, will nurse you? Whoever, O *bhikkhus*, would nurse me, he should nurse the sick."[164] The reason for this lecture was that a monk who had fallen seriously ill with a bowel disturbance had not been taken care of by his fellow monks. The reluctance of the monks to nurse him is described as being due to his uselessness to them rather than to the repulsive nature of his disease. However, the Buddha's further admonitions show that the often repugnant nature of nursing was probably at the heart of the conflict after all:

> The qualities of a competent nurse to the sick are as follows: he is competent to provide medicine; he knows what is beneficial and nonbeneficial; he offers what is beneficial and takes away what is nonbeneficial; he nurses the sick with a kindly thought, not out of greed; *he is not unwilling to remove feces, urine, mucus, or vomit*; and he is competent to gladden, rejoice, rouse, and delight the sick from time to time with a story about Buddhist doctrine [*dhamma*].[165]

This story provides an answer to the question who in normal society, outside the Buddhist monks' community, would have taken up the role of the attendant: a family member. Being a nurse or attendant, then, would not have been a professional occupation but a role taken up by relatives as and when necessary. This scenario, however, stands somewhat uneasily with what Caraka suggests should be the attendant's characteristics: knowledge of attendance and skill.[166] And Kaśyapa's list of requirements, which emphasizes experience and knowledge—professional skills, in other words—would be asking rather a lot of an amateur. Caraka's "knowledge of attendance" (*upacārajñatā*) may of course not encompass very complicated medical skills. According to Cakrapāṇidatta, it means "knowing how to prepare soups and juices, how to soothe a person to sleep through massage, and so on,"[167] which should be possible to achieve without specialist training. However, these very tasks are listed in another context as work for employees, as we will see. More significantly, Suśruta and Kaśyapa speak of the relationship between physician and attendant as one between master and subordinate. Suśruta notes that the attendant should be obedient to the physician, while Kaśyapa demands the attendant's devotion to his master. Since we learn nothing of an attendant's training from the medical classics, and since there is also no mention of attendants working independently of physicians, we cannot assume nursing to have been an actual profession. It is more likely that medical attendants were servants of the physician, albeit with some specialist skills. This is also the conclusion Leslie and Wujastyk (1991, 27–28) come to:

> It is clear from rulings like these that the doctor had to organize his own practice or dispensary, from the physical aspects of the house or room and the instruments and facilities within it to the nursing staff or attendants who helped him care for the sick. It is also clear that, while these attendants had a specialized function within the doctor's entourage, they were in fact his personal servants or employees, and that they were dependent on the doctor for their board as well as for their training.

However, there is also the possibility that the patients' servants or, in the case of the king as patient, close members of his court may have performed the service of attendants. In Sū.15, Caraka describes complex preparations for a particular type of medical treatment (purgation and emesis) for the king or aristocratic or rich persons,[168] which included the selection of suitable attendants:

> After that, one should select the staff of soup and rice cooks, bath attendants, masseurs [*saṃvāhaka*], people to help patients with getting up and sitting down, and herb grinders. They should be good-natured, clean, well-behaved, loyal, practical, and pious. They should be skilled in nursing, and accomplished in all treatments. They should not be reluctant to work. The attendants should be able to sing, play instruments, and perform recitations, as well as being skilled in verses, songs, stories, legends, and ancient lore. They should be pleasant and able to

anticipate. They should know the where and when of things, and be generally sociable.[169]

From this description, it would seem that the therapy room was a fairly busy place with a whole entourage of staff to perform a variety of tasks, many of them aimed at entertaining the patient. This makes sense in regard to the high status of the patient, who is likely to expect special attention. And the nature of the therapy may allow for a certain amount of fun and games in between treatments: Emesis and purgation can be administered to healthy patients as part of a preventative or rejuvenative regime rather than to counteract an illness. As part of the former, these treatments would be comparable to what would now be spa therapies, and a patient, while in need of rest, would still be able to enjoy entertainment. Thus, many of the attendants' required qualifications are basically entertainment skills needed for diverting the patient's attention from any discomfort and for dispelling his ennui. Caraka summarizes preparations for this therapy as follows: "Whatever other means one might procure in addition to what has been listed above to prevent complications and to give pleasure should be arranged."[170] While this quote refers to equipment rather than to people, its division into medicine ("complications") and entertainment ("pleasure") can still be applied to the attendants' tasks. It is tempting to postulate two types of attendants: those who take care of the more menial or specifically medical chores (herb grinders, cooks, bath attendants) and thus help medical treatment run smoothly, and those who provide stimulating company (musicians, actors, and storytellers) and thus ensure a comfortable and generally positive experience. Such a division in tasks could also have mirrored a division in attendants' provenance: Medical problems could be taken care of by the physician's specialist servants, entertainment by the rich man's servants or, in the case of the king, by his court entourage. However, from Caraka's description it would appear that he envisioned his ideal attendant as an all-around talent: literally an all-singing, all-dancing nurse.

An inscription on the Viṣṇu temple of Veṅkateśa–Perumāḷ at Tirumukkūḍal from about the ninth century paints a different picture: It records salaries for medical personnel who staffed a hospital (*āturaśālā*) sponsored by the South Indian king of the Cola dynasty, Rājakeśarivarman. According to the inscription, staff included a surgeon, two persons for gathering medicinal herbs and firewood and preparing the medicines, two nurses to attend the patients and administer the medicines, and a barber.[171] While there is no mention of singers, dancers, or storytellers, the inscription does provide clear evidence for a division of labor between those who prepared medicines and those who dealt with patients directly.

While definitions of the four pillars of medicine create the image that a medical setting is complete if it includes a physician, a patient, medicine, and an attendant, the medical treatises also offer a more complicated picture of medical treatment in which the four pillars are complemented by other persons who contribute in various ways to medical practice. These include cooks and kitchen staff, friends of the patient, midwives and experienced women who aid at births, wet-nurses (who are particularly singled out in the *Kāśyapasaṃhitā*), and persons able to provide information about medicinal plants, such as cowherds and goatherds, hunters, forest-dwellers, and hermits. Though these additional helpers are not mentioned in connection with the four pillars of treatment, they appear in other contexts and are there described as an important part of medical care.

Kitchen staff. While Caraka mentions soup and rice cooks as part of special arrangements for emesis and purgation therapy in Ca.Sū.15.7, Suśruta gives quite detailed instructions on regular staff for the royal kitchens, including a physician and a supervisor to oversee the assistants:

> The kitchens ... should be staffed by qualified men and women. And someone who has most of the same virtues as a doctor should be appointed as supervisor.
>
> There should be various assistants who are clean, competent, expert, well-behaved and nice-looking. They should be very loyal, cheerful, dependable, and have short hair and nails. They should have washed, and be firmly self-disciplined, with their hair back in a bunch, restrained, and obedient when instructed.
>
> Living beings depend on food, so the doctor should be very conscientious where the kitchens are concerned. The kitchen staff, including bearers, chefs for the soups, puddings, and cakes, and whoever else may be there, must all be under the strict control of the doctor.[172]

These kitchen arrangements were meant to ensure the king's safety in regard to poisoning, be it food poisoning or intentional attempts to poison the king. The hierarchy in the kitchen, with two heads of staff, is interesting, though it is not clear how the roles of the physician and of the supervisor differ from each other. Since the supervisor should be as like the physician as possible, the difference of position between the two may reflect not a division in tasks but only one in rank.

Friends. Establishing hierarchy between the physician, the primary carers, and auxiliary staff seems to have been deemed essential in the professional setup of medical care. Caraka, however, seems to also allow for relationships outside this tightly controlled hierarchy in the sickroom. He describes the presence of friends (*suhṛd*), or at least of kindhearted persons who are there to provide emotional comfort with their tender loving care: "Loving friends, who should be unembarrassed, may help in holding his forehead and supporting his sides, pressing his navel, and rubbing his back".[173] We cannot be sure that *suhṛd* means a friend here rather than a kindhearted attendant (who would be subject to the aforementioned hierarchy), since kindness is required of attendants by at least two of the medical authors: Suśruta describes his perfect attendant as loving (*snigdha*) and Vāgbhaṭa's attendant is affectionate (*anurakta*).[174] Whether friends or friendly help, these persons obviously provide a crucial service to the patient. The fact that their presence is described as part of how such a treatment should be undertaken shows that giving comfort to a patient was seen as an intrinsic part of therapy.

Midwives and experienced women. The question of comfort and support appears in another context: at the delivery house (*sūtikāgāra*). This setting is a complete departure from the usual medical scene, in which all persons involved—the physician, the attendant, and the patient—are male. At the delivery house, women are at the center of action: the woman who is about to give birth and the women who are assisting her. The latter do not seem to be professional midwives but simply friendly women who have given birth to several children themselves and thus are experienced in the matters of childbirth. Caraka describes them thus in Śā.8.34:

> And there should be women, many women who have repeatedly given birth, who are yoked with good-heartedness, constantly attentive, who have respectful manners, are clever in resources, who are loving mothers by nature, who have put aside disgust, who can endure pain, and who are loved by others.[175]

These women provide practical help and give advice regarding arrangements in the delivery house as well as to the laboring woman. Their authority is such that, in this instance, their advice is put on par with that of the brahmins whose services are also needed at the delivery house: "There should also be brahmins who know the *Atharvaveda*, and whatever other thing might be thought suitable in this situation. Whatever other things the brahmins and elderly women might say, that should be done".[176] The experienced women verbally coach the woman who is about to give birth (probably for the first time, as Selby [2005, 271] argues) through the birthing process.

Caraka describes the comfort the attending women provide:

> And at the appearance of birth pangs, one should arrange a bed on the ground and outfit it with soft linens. She should sit on it. Then, surrounding her completely, women with the characteristics as stated should attend on her, consoling her with appropriate and soothing words.[177]

They murmur blessings into her ears, and accompany the moment of birth with chants. Selby (2005, 273) suggests that the protection the surrounding women offer goes both ways: they protect the laboring woman from the eyes of the brahmins (and possibly of the physician, though it is not quite clear whether he is present at the birth at all) and the brahmins from her. However, Caraka does not describe any further actions of the brahmins after they have given their blessings at the time the pregnant woman enters the delivery house. There seems to be no interaction during labor or after the birth. And given that the woman is to enter the delivery house at the beginning of the ninth month of her pregnancy to wait for labor to begin—which can take days, if not weeks—it seems unlikely (though not impossible) that these brahmins are meant to wait around to be present for the birth proper.

Caraka's vivid account is paralleled by Suśruta with a similar, though perhaps slightly less evocative, description in Śā.10.8. There, the attending women are briefly described as follows: "Four reliable women who are advanced in age and skilled in midwifery, and whose nails are cut short, should attend to her." Somewhat surprisingly, the woman who is about to give birth is also to be surrounded by boys (*kumāraparivṛtā*). Their presence may be required to influence the gender of the child to be born, in a similar symbolic way to the fruit with masculine names that the laboring woman is meant to hold in her hands.[178] The theme of the attending women providing comfort and protection to the laboring woman, so central to Caraka's birthing scene, is hardly touched on by Suśruta. His keywords—reliability, skill, and having short nails—evoke brisk professionalism rather than motherly and empathetic attendance.

Wet-nurses. The medical authors describe one further person involved in medical care: the wet-nurse. She is a fairly central character in Kaśyapa's compendium, where a whole chapter is dedicated to her (Cik.18). The wet-nurse's role is dual: she is both a patient and a carer. The person she cares for—the baby—is not necessarily ill, but it is her own health and aptitude for the task of feeding that are the foundation of the child's health and well-being. Her work, a task of love, takes its toll on her, according to Kaśyapa: "The wet-nurse suffers the draining of her own body for the sake of the son's body, and many other terrible afflictions out of love."[179]

Suśruta has a whole list of characteristics a wet-nurse should fulfill:

> Then one should approach the wet-nurse, who, for the health, strength, and growth of the child, should be of the same class (*varṇa*), of medium height, middle-aged, healthy, well-behaved, steady, free from desire, neither obese, nor too thin. Her milk should be clear, her lips not large, her breasts should neither be pendulous nor high. She should be not deformed, and free from evil practices. Her children should be alive, and she should be lactating and child-loving. She should not act in a low manner. She should come from a good family and therefore she should possess abundant good qualities, and should be of dark complexion.[180]

Caraka offers a strikingly similar list of wet-nurse characteristics in Śā.8.52. His list is in fact given as a quote, so it seems likely that he and Suśruta used the same source. There are some minor differences: Where Suśruta demands that the wet-nurse should have living children (*jīvadvatsā*), Caraka adds that she should have male offspring (*puṃvatsā*). Caraka also makes much of the wet-nurse's cleanliness and purity, in terms of both hygiene and class. She should not be of a low caste (*anantyāvasāyinī*), and she should be clean and abhor what is unclean.

Those who know plants. Finally, the medical authors mention persons who aid the physician in his work by giving him information on plant materials needed for his medicines: goatherds, shepherds, cowherds, hunters, hermits, and other forest-dwellers.[181] Their contribution to medical care lies in helping the physician identify plants, which they know by name and form. Caraka is quick to point out that while they may know which plant is which, they do not know how to use them medicinally. That is solely the domain of the physician. He, on the other hand, may not be able to identify the plants. Still, even if the physician only knows the plants' application, he is a "knower of truth," and indeed, knowing plants in every respect makes him the very best of physicians. Those who can identify plants function as repositories of useful, though limited, knowledge. The exchange between them and the physician seems to happen as part of his general stocking up with equipment. As they do not participate directly in treatments, they are not really part of the medical team, as it were, but play an important role in the background.

To conclude, despite all the textual material, it is difficult to tease out an actual ethic of nursing from these descriptions. We get a glimpse into what a medical attendant (or a wet-nurse) should be like: obedient to the physician, kind to the patient, and ready and able to do the job. Conversely, we know what an attendant should not be like: A bad attendant would be vulgar, dirty, badly behaved, disloyal, impractical, and impious. He would be unskilled in nursing, unaccomplished in all treatments, and reluctant to work. This does not, however, bring us much closer to an idea of the dos and don'ts of medical attendance. The characteristics the medical authors describe seem more like selection criteria that the physician should heed when setting up his medical team. The question of what behavior might be grounds for dismissal is not touched on. Neither are we offered any insight into moral conflicts that nursing might present to an attendant. We do not learn much about an attendant's actions during treatment, or about his interactions with the patient (Caraka's "friend" (*suhṛd*) is the exception to this rule). And since there is no description of an attendant's actions, there is also no moral evaluation of them. One reason for this may be that the medical authors envisage the attendant as absolutely subordinate to and dependent on the physician, with no agency or will of his own. Nothing he does is done on his own initiative; he merely follows the physician's orders. It is as if the attendant were a physical extension of the physician, his unthinking hired hand, applying and thus embodying some of the physician's theoretical knowledge. Yet intelligence and knowledge are described as the attendant's prerequisites in the four-pillar definitions, so perhaps his work entailed more agency and hence more moral choice than can be inferred from the descriptions available from the medical classics.

2

On Becoming a Physician

A MEDICAL STUDENT'S education and his subsequent entry into the medical profession are outlined in several of the ayurvedic classics: in Ca.Vi.8, in Su.Sū.2–4 (with additional relevant passages in Su.Sū.9.3 and 10.3–4, and 9), and in As.Sū.2.1–20.[182] There is also relevant material in what has been preserved of the Vimānasthāna of the *Kāśyapasaṃhitā* (in the chapter entitled "*Śiṣyopakramaṇīya*") and in the first chapter of the *Hārītasaṃhitā*. According to Preisendanz (2007, 630), there is some reason to believe that the *Bhelasaṃhitā* may have contained some text on the medical student's education on the basis of its special relationship with the *Carakasaṃhitā*, but Preisendanz concludes that this must remain a matter of speculation in view of its fragmentary transmission. Of the above texts, Caraka's rendition of the procedures of medical studies is the most complex and comprehensive, and as such will be used as the blueprint for discussion. It is particularly useful to do so in view of its presenting the themes of medical education in one coherent chapter. I broadly follow the order in which Caraka introduces and develops these themes, comparing them to the other author's versions.[183]

The Preliminaries of Medical Education

Identifying the Best Materials for Study

Caraka begins his discussion of the preliminaries of medical education with advice to the aspiring student on how to choose a suitable medical work for study.

> A discerning person who wants to become a physician should start by selecting a text based on a consideration of his ability to cope with hard or easy tasks, the results he is after, the likely aftermath, the place and the time. After all, there are numerous physicians' manuals in circulation in the world, so he should apply himself only to a text which is extremely famous, which is used by scholars, which covers a lot of topics, and is respected by qualified people. It has to be good for pupils of

> all three levels of ability, and it should not be flawed by repetitiousness. It should be derived from the tradition of the saints. The sequence of its text, commentary, and summary should be well organized. It should be solidly based, and have no corrupt or missing words. It should be full of significance, its ideas should follow in sequence and it should give importance to determining the truth about things. Its ideas should be coherent, and its topics should not be haphazard. It should communicate its meaning rapidly, and it should have both definitions and examples. This type of text is like a flawless sun: it dispels darkness and throws light on everything.[184]

This passage has also been partly translated and commented on by Scharfe (2002, 258) and Preisendanz (2007, 639). Their understanding of the beginning of the passage differs from Wujastyk's interpretation. In Wujastyk's translation, the student evaluates his own needs and abilities in order to choose a suitable textbook (or body of knowledge) for study. By contrast, both Scharfe and Preisendanz understand the student's self-evaluation to be related to his ability and suitability for the study of medicine and its subsequent practice in general. That is, before embarking on the study of medicine, a person should think hard about whether he is suited to the tasks of the profession at all. Preisendanz writes that "only then he should proceed to critically examine various bodies of medical knowledge."[185]

We find elsewhere passages in which the physician is encouraged to engage in critical self-reflection. For example, in Ca.Vi.8.86, the former medical student has already entered the profession, but must ask himself whether he is capable of carrying out the work or not before undertaking a procedure. The self-questioning that comes before any action is one of the markers that show him to be a good physician, since "the experts commend the undertaking of actions to be preceded by knowledge."[186]

Although Scharfe's and Preisendanz's interpretation of the first sentence makes sense in the larger scheme of the chapter, and can also be justified in terms of grammar, in my view Wujastyk's rendering makes more sense in terms of the sentence's structure and immediate context. It seems odd, after all, to casually introduce as important a theme as the student's self-reflection in regard to his future as a physician as part of a sentence about choosing a treatise for study that itself is placed within a passage devoted to defining a good textbook.

It is somewhat surprising that Caraka would have the student—rather than his teacher—choose a textbook that suits his needs and abilities in the first place. While Caraka provides guidelines on how to recognize a good textbook—it should be famous, its ideas should be introduced in a logical sequence, and so on—the likelihood of a novice to the field arriving at a suitable choice seems doubtful. One would rather expect a teacher to make an informed choice of suitable teaching materials for a student. This scenario of a nonspecialist being required to display relevant knowledge and discernment appears several times in the medical classics. Remember, for example, the patient in Kaśyapa's four-pillar definition who is full of exact and comprehensive information on his medical condition for the physician. Or Caraka's and Suśruta's patients who are required to be knowledgeable enough to know when a doctor is a genuine physician and when he is a quack.[187] Knowledgeable and discerning patients may arrive at their judgments through natural intelligence and common sense. The medical-student-to-be needs more solid means of acquiring initial knowledge: book learning. He must be able to read and to understand the contents of what he is reading. He must also be aware of what literature is available in the field and must have the means to get hold of whatever literature there is. This all points to his being a scholar with previous learning who is conversant in the methods of critical study.

However, apparently this does not mean that the student must be a paragon of knowledge. After all, one of the markers of a suitable textbook is that "it has to be good for pupils of all three levels of ability."[188] Cakrapāṇidatta explains these three kinds of pupils to be those of great, moderate, and little intelligence.[189] This is an interesting point, since Caraka elsewhere notes that a chapter is written in such a way that will make it accessible to those of little intelligence, while those with greater intelligence will be able to infer further and more profound information from its contents.[190] In other words, his treatise fulfills the requirement of being suitable to students of all levels. Suśruta, on the other hand, emphasizes the role of the teacher in interpreting his work, since the ideas presented in it are subtle, and "baffle even the mind of one of pure and great intelligence, let alone one of little intelligence."[191] Compare this with Śārṅgadhara's outright admission that his work is aimed at the less clever: "This book has been composed with the power of giving short-lived, dim-witted people the benefit of reading the entire canon. So study this work diligently for your own good: it collects in one place just the bare essentials."[192]

Finally, Caraka's statement that "there are numerous physicians' manuals in circulation in the world" is interesting for various reasons. The use of the word *śāstra*, which Wujastyk has translated as "text" and as "manual," is worth discussing. Caraka seems to be describing an actual physical object rather than an abstract body of knowledge. He notes, for example, that a text should "have no corrupt or missing words"—more likely to apply to a written text than a memorized one. This changes the classroom scene from one in which the teacher lectures the student without using written materials to one in which the teacher reads from a manuscript, or even one in which the teacher and student pore over a text together. (The student must, after all, be able to read, since he is required to pass judgement on medical manuals prior to his studies with the teacher.) The difference between book learning and oral tradition may, however, be quite slight, if the subject of oral transmission is a composed text that has been memorized. And indeed, the method of study Caraka describes in Vi.8.7 is one of memorizing aphorisms through repeated recitation.

By mentioning "numerous physicians' manuals in circulation in the world," Caraka creates the impression of a lively medical world in his times, with an established literature (though of varying quality). Note, however, that Caraka does not recommend any particular works or name any specific topics that must be included in the ideal medical manual. His main criteria concern the manual's inner structure, its logic, and the way ideas are presented in it. These requirements could be applied to any body of knowledge, not just to medicine, and we cannot deduce a partisanship to any lineage of learning from them—not even to his own.

Choosing the Teacher

Caraka follows his description of how to choose a good textbook with one of how to choose a teacher. While most of the medical classics have something to say about what makes someone eligible as a student, only Caraka and Kaśyapa write about what characteristics a student should look for in a prospective teacher. Caraka writes in Vi.8.4:

> Next, one should examine the teacher according to whether he is accomplished in the discipline and has observed practice extensively, whether he is skilled, competent, and clean, whether his hands are trained, whether he has all the (necessary) equipment, whether he has his wits about him, knows about natural states and about procedures, whether his knowledge is flawless, whether he is free from self-conceit, envy, or anger, whether he is capable of enduring distress,[193] whether he is affectionate toward his students, and a teacher who is capable of imparting knowledge. Such a teacher quickly furnishes a good student with the qualities of a physician the way a seasonable cloud furnishes a good field with the qualities of grain.

These characteristics divide into those pertaining to the teacher's competence as a physician and those pertaining more directly to his didactic abilities as a teacher. The former are well known to us from other passages on the good physician: knowledge and skill.[194] The physician as a teacher must fulfill further requirements: He must be capable of transmitting what he knows, and he must also be affectionately committed to his students. Kaśyapa's take on this is similar:

> Now the preceptor: He is one whose expertise includes virtue, knowledge, discernment, comprehension, reasoning, and perception, who is endowed with good qualities, who is pleasant to look at and clean, a teacher who teaches for the student's benefit, skilled at explaining the medical works, whose knowledge and understanding come from a preceptor, who is healthy, has no other commitments and [whose attention is] undivided, and who has the [same] qualities as the student. Otherwise he should be avoided because of his being defective.[195]

This not only stresses didactic abilities but positions a teacher's commitment to his student—giving him full and undivided attention, and always having his best interests at heart—at the center of a good teacher's defining characteristics.

Both Caraka's and Kaśyapa's descriptions of the good teacher are written from the perspective of the student: rather than telling a physician what he should be like as a teacher, they explain to the student searching for a teacher what he should look for. Caraka writes; "one should examine the teacher," and so on, and follows his list of desirable characteristics with instructions on how to proceed once one has identified a suitable teacher: "Having approached him, one who wishes to please him should serve him attentively like a fire, a god, a king, a father, or a master".[196] Kaśyapa offers no such advice but concludes his passage with the warning that a teacher who does not fulfill the criteria mentioned should be avoided.[197] It thus seems that both authors envisage the student's participation in selecting a teacher to be active and informed, similar to his choosing the body of knowledge that is to provide the foundation of his studies.

Undertaking Studies

Caraka follows his description of how to choose a teacher with an excursion on the method of study.[198] In Vi.8.5–6, Caraka defines studying, teaching, and discussion with experts as the means for "a firm [grasp] of the discipline, an excellent [command] of its terminology, an understanding of its theories, and the ability to relate [them]."[199]

In the next passage (Ca.Vi.8.7), he explains in detail how one should undertake study:

> Ready and impatient [to study], one should get up at daybreak or about dawn. Having done what is necessary, one should sip water and pay homage to the gods, sages, cows, brahmins, preceptors, elders, accomplished persons, and the teacher.[200] Sitting comfortably on an even and pure spot, one should recite the treatise again and again, going through it in order, first mentally, then out loud.[201] After one has understood and properly entered into the true meaning [of the treatise], one should thus constantly practice, studying at noon, in the afternoon, and at night without omission, in order to avoid mistakes of one's own and to judge the mistakes of others.[202]

Caraka emphasizes two aspects of study. The first is the formal setup of study: that study should start in a ritualistic way by paying homage to the gods, and so on, and that the student should sit in a certain manner in a certain place. The second aspect of study concerns its methodology: learning by rote. Caraka stresses the need to put effort and time into learning practice, and suggests the use of repetition for memorizing and understanding relevant knowledge.

Suśruta provides similar instructions in Sū.3.54–55. The main difference from Caraka's description is that Suśruta describes the interaction between teacher (or preceptor) and student:

> The preceptor should teach a student who is clean and has put on an upper garment, who is untroubled, and who has presented himself at the [prescribed] time of study according to his ability a word, a quarter verse, or a verse. And these words, quarter verses, and verses should moreover be set in order again and again. In this way, he should bring them together one by one. And he should repeat [them] by himself neither too quickly, nor too slowly, without hesitation, not speaking through the nose, enunciating the syllables well, without slurring the sounds, without embellishing with his eyes, eyebrows, lips, or hands, and correctly. He should read in a voice that is neither too high, nor too low. And no one should pass between the two while they study. On this, there are [these verses]: A student who is clean, who is devoted to the teacher, able, free from laziness and sloth, and who studies according to this method should reach the limits of the discipline.

Suśruta's description is a little unclear in regard to who is doing what at which time. Following the sequence of events (that is, "The teacher should teach a student ... a word, etc.," and then "He should repeat [*anupaṭhet*] them"), it seems likely that the teacher is meant to recite the words/lines/verses first and the student is then meant to repeat them. Ḍalhaṇa, however, would have it the other way around, explaining that the teacher recites after the student in order to improve the student's recitation.[203] If Ḍalhaṇa's interpretation is correct, then we must assume that teacher and student are reading out loud from a manuscript (rather than that the student is memorizing the teacher's words). The teacher's role, then, is to correct the student's pronunciation, making sure he reads well. In both cases, the aim of the lesson in general seems to be for the student to memorize the text (hence the reading or reciting word by word, or stanza by stanza). Elsewhere, as noted, Suśruta explains the teacher's role as lying in the interpretation of the texts, arguing that a student cannot understand the contents of a treatise by himself, since the ideas presented in it are subtle, and "baffle even the mind of one of pure and great intelligence, let alone one of little intelligence."[204] Though this is part of another chapter, it follows on more or less directly from Su.Sū.3.54, linked by the statement that

> reading, that, though completed, has not been clarified in regard to its meaning just becomes wearying, as carrying sandalwood is wearying to a donkey. In regard to this there is [this verse]: Just as a donkey carrying a load of sandalwood experiences the load but not the sandalwood, those who have studied many treatises and are ignorant of their meaning feel like the donkey.[205]

Preisendanz (2007, 645) notes that "there is one theme that is curiously absent in the *Carakasaṃhitā* in the present context, but treated rather extensively by Suśruta and Kaśyapa, namely the times and occasions when study has to be discontinued or should not be taken up at all (*anadhyāya*)."[206] The medical authors' prescriptions in regard to suitable times for study broadly conform to parallel directions given in *dharma* literature, according to Preisendanz.[207]

Finally, Suśruta emphasizes the importance of developing manual skills, suggesting that students should practice surgery on vegetables, and so on.[208] This fits in well with the generally pervasive idea that a good doctor should be not only versed in theory but also skilled in practice.

Choosing the Student

Following the excursion on the method of study, Caraka gives advice to the teacher on how to choose a student.[209] The good student is a topic on which several of the medical authors have something to say. Suśruta, Vāgbhaṭa, Kaśyapa, and Hārīta all give guidelines on how to identify who is suitable to study medicine and who is not. Caraka's list of desired traits is the longest:

> A teacher who is resolved to teach should first observe the pupil according to whether he is calm and noble-natured, whether his actions are not vulgar, whether his eyes, mouth, and nasal bridge are straight, his tongue is thin, red, and clear, and his teeth and lips are well-shaped, whether he does not speak through the nose, is resolute and free from self-conceit, whether he is intelligent, endowed with deliberation and mindfulness and generous-minded, whether he comes from a family of physicians, or else behaves as such, whether he is devoted to truth, without deformity, his senses unimpaired, modest, and humble, whether his opinion is authoritative [*arthattvabhāvaka*],[210] whether he is without anger and free from vice, whether he has a good character, pure habits, affection, and skill and behaves respectfully, whether he wishes to study and has no other aim than to understand theory and practice, whether he is not avaricious or lazy, strives for the welfare of all beings, follows all the teacher's instructions, and loves [studying or the teacher]:[211] One with such qualities is considered fit to be taught.

The characteristics Caraka describes divide into those pertaining to physical appearance (straight mouth, thin tongue, etc.); to character or personality (generosity, resoluteness, etc.), attitudes (respect toward the teacher, devotion to work and to patients), and behavior (not acting in a vulgar way, etc.); to social background (coming from a family of physicians, etc.); and finally to cognitive abilities. The traits relating to the student's physical appearance may be connected to his social background but may also only reflect aesthetic preferences. A good physician, as defined in the various four-pillar definitions, is mainly characterized by his knowledge and skill, and much emphasis is given to his cognitive abilities. A student has not yet acquired the set of skills and the store of knowledge that a physician should have command of. However, Caraka would have his student "intelligent" and "endowed with deliberation and mindfulness," with "his senses unimpaired." In other words, a student should be able to understand and digest the information given to him by the teacher. He is also required to be extremely devoted to his studies and to his teacher: The ideal student "wishes to study and has no other aim than to understand theory and practice," and lastly he "follows all the teacher's instructions" and loves him (or loves studying). Coming from a physician's family, or behaving as such, implies a familiarity with the "tricks of the trade"—its customs and etiquette, but perhaps also some prior knowledge of pharmacopoeia and treatment methods.

The other traits make the student a pleasant person to be around: good looks and good behavior are a powerful combination in any social situation.

Interestingly, characteristics pertaining to physical appearance or behavior are not generally listed as the physician's basic virtues in the four-pillar definitions of Caraka, Suśruta, and Vāgbhaṭa, though they are part of Kaśyapa's definition of perfection in a physician. A physician's physical appearance and behavior are, however, described at length by Caraka, Suśruta, and Vāgbhaṭa in their descriptions of the medical student's initiation or his entry into the profession. Caraka's model student, then, is an agreeable companion, easy and gratifying to teach, and already halfway on his path to becoming part of an intellectual elite.

Suśruta has a slightly different take on the question of the student's social background. He declares that a "physician should initiate any brahmin, someone from the ruling classes [*kṣatriya*], or someone from the trade classes [*vaiśya*] from a good family,"[212] which leaves the profession open to all but *śūdras* (members of the serving classes). Suśruta then, however, notes that "according to some," *śūdras* may in fact be initiated into the profession, albeit without using mantras at the ceremony.[213] The use of "according to some," on the other hand, points to this being an unusual practice, known to Suśruta by hearsay rather than from common occurrence. Another feature stands out in Suśruta's delineation: among the virtues a student should display are strength and vigor, courage, and being equal to distress. The latter could be understood in two ways: being equal to experiencing one's own distress or to experiencing someone else's suffering, for example the patient's during surgery. None of these virtues occur in the other authors' descriptions of the student's characteristics. However, Suśruta lists similar ones for his ideal physician in his four-pillar definition, where the emphasis is on physical abilities, particularly light-handedness, swiftness, and strength, and their psychological counterparts, readiness of mind and resolve. I have noted that this probably reflects the specific medical context of surgery as opposed to general practice. The same principle applies to an apprenticeship in surgery.

The *Aṣṭāṅgahṛdayasaṃhitā* omits any description of medical education; the *Aṣṭāṅgasaṃgraha* gives an abbreviated version in Sū.2.2–4ab.[214] Its description of the eligible medical student covers the same points as the *Carakasaṃhitā*. Its only notable addition is that it speaks of a period of six months in which the student proves himself to the teacher. It is not entirely clear from the text whether this is a probational period, after which the teacher decides whether he will take on the student for good, or a more informal period of a teacher watching a potential student before commencing any sort of class with him.

The *Kāśyapasaṃhitā* also follows the general pattern found in the *Carakasaṃhitā*, with somewhat greater emphasis on the virtues of gentle and nonviolent behavior.[215] Suśruta and Kaśyapa concur in stating that whoever does not fulfill the named positive requirements should not be taught. Caraka says something similar at the end of his description of the student's initiation in Vi.8.14: "If he acts according to these instructions, he should be taught, otherwise, however, he should not be taught." However, this pertains not just to a student's eligibility but also to the time when a student has already been accepted.

The sole contribution of the *Hārītasaṃhitā* on the subject of student eligibility concerns whom not to teach: those who are not devoted (*abhakta*), not calm (*aśānta*), stupid (*mūrkha*), or lowly (*adhama*).[216]

The characteristics listed by the medical authors that qualify or disqualify a person from becoming a student are not dissimilar to those known to us from earlier texts of *smṛti* literature. According to Yāska's Nirukta (2.4), the teacher was to avoid teaching a student who "was jealous (or who treated *vidyā* with contempt), was crooked and was not self–restrained."[217] Conversely, a student who was "pure, attentive, intelligent and endowed with brahmacarya [celibacy], who would never prove false [to his teacher] and who would guard what he learnt as a treasure" was eligible.[218] *Manusmṛti* (2.109 and 112) gives a list of ten persons deserving of being taught the Veda:

> The son of his teacher, a person who offers obedient service, a person who has given him knowledge, a virtuous person, an honest person, someone close to him, a capable man, someone who gives him money, a good man, and one who is his own.[219]

Manu warns not to impart knowledge to those who have not requested to be taught, or who have requested it in an improper way (2.111). He states more generally that teaching should not be undertaken "where there is no merit or money, or at least proportionate service" (2.112).[220] Yājñavalkyasmṛti 1.28 reiterates Manu's list and adds that "the student must be grateful, not inclined to hate or prove false to the teacher, healthy and not disposed to find fault."[221] The similarities to the medical authors' requirements of the student are striking. Manu's stress on money stands out as an exception—none of the medical authors mention a student's ability to pay his teacher. The other difference between the medical treatise's treatment of the subject and that of the *smṛtis* is the former's requirements regarding the student's physique. A final but crucial difference between them is the question of the student's social background. The *smṛtis* deal with the study of Vedic knowledge, which they define as the prerogative, indeed the duty, of every twice-born person.[222] This means that the study of the Vedas was open to and required of brahmins, *kṣatriyas*, and *vaiśyas* but denied to *śūdras*. As we have seen, among the medical authors only Suśruta makes mention of the student's class background (*varṇa*), and he does not rule out that *śūdras* may be taught. For the other medical authors, the question of social background (in terms of class, *varṇa*, at least) does not seem to feature in this context.

The teacher's choice of student mirrors the student's choice of teacher. Both are based as much on their mutual suitability as persons who will live together closely during the apprenticeship as on their suitability for their respective tasks of teaching and of studying. The responsibility for laying the foundations of a successful apprenticeship thus lies equally in both the student's and the teacher's hands from the beginning.

How the actual search for a teacher or student was handled on a practical level, however, is left to our imagination. Caraka's description in Vi.8.5 of the student approaching the teacher seems to happen at the end of an informal evaluation process, in which both teacher and student work out whether they are suitable for each other. Perhaps the student finds out about the teacher first, and is then subject to the teacher's scrutiny once he has approached him. However, neither Caraka nor Kaśyapa (or the other authors) offers a chronology of the events, and the order in which descriptions of student and teacher eligibility occur in the texts is not enough to give certainty on how this would have happened. The impression one gets from reading the relevant passages, however, is that the initial selection process is informal and not subject to any form of application process. The next step in actually commencing medical studies, on the other hand, takes place in a formalized procedure: the medical student's initiation.

The Initiation of the Medical Student

As noted, the passage in the *Carakasaṃhitā* that describes the initiation of the medical student[223] has been the subject matter of a number of studies and in fact was one of the earliest text passages in the Sanskrit medical classics to be translated and commented on.[224] The most recent and most thorough of these studies is the article by Preisendanz,[225] which not only gives a structural analysis of Ca.Vi.8 but also provides a comparative table of the corresponding (as well as additionally relevant) passages in the *Suśrutasaṃhitā* and the *Kāśyapasaṃhitā*. Her analyses have enabled Preisendanz to make three conclusions. First, the segment on the initiation of the student is a genuine part of the *Carakasaṃhitā* and is well integrated into the intellectual world of the medical tradition as reflected in the treatise, while also showing much resemblance to descriptions of the student's initiation in the Dharmaśāstras. Second, the treatment of the topic in the *Carakasaṃhitā* closely resembles those in the

Suśrutasaṃhitā and the *Kāśyapasaṃhitā*, though all three texts also "exhibit considerable differences from the points of view of structure, wording, content and orientation of the exposition."[226] Third, Kaśyapa attaches himself more closely to Caraka than to Suśruta.

Preisendanz offers two structural overviews of Caraka's passage on the medical student's initiation. The first is part of her analysis of the whole of Vimānasthāna 8[227] and is a fairly concise categorization of the passage's contents. The second is part of her comparative structural analysis of Ca.Vi.8.3–67 and the corresponding passages in the *Suśrutasaṃhitā* and the *Kāśyapasaṃhitā* and gives summaries of the contents of each respective passage.[228] From the first overview, we learn that the initiation proper begins in *sūtra* 11 and is part of a section on teaching (itself a subcategory to a wider passage spanning Ca.Vi.8.5–151 that Preisendanz entitles "Becoming a Physician").[229] The initiation is preceded by the teacher deciding to take up teaching, and instructing his prospective student to bring certain items in preparation for the initiation ceremony in Ca.Vi.8.9–10:

> When such a pupil, eager to learn and wishing to gain [his] favor, has presented himself, the teacher should address him [as follows]: "In the half year from the winter to the summer solstice, in the bright half of the month, on an auspicious day, when the venerable moon has entered into a conjunction with either the constellation *tiṣya*, *hasta*, *śravaṇa*, or *aśvayuj*, in the most auspicious part of the day,[230] at a favorable moment,[231] having shaved your head, having fasted and bathed, wearing an orange garment and with scented hands, you should give offerings of firewood, fire, clarified butter, paste, water vessels, garlands, wreaths, lamps, gold, golden objects,[232] silver, precious stones, pearls, corals, silk, sticks for enclosing the sacrificial fire [*paridhi*], *kuśa* grass,[233] parched rice, mustard seeds, and unbroken grains; white flowers,[234] strung together, or loose, intellect-promoting foods and ground sandalwood." He should do it accordingly.

The information the teacher gives the student here concerns (1) the right times for the initiation, (2) the correct attire and appearance for presenting himself, and (3) the items to bring to the ceremony.

The Right Times

Caraka's recommendations (or prescriptions) regarding proper times for initiation are quite vague, particularly in regard to the time of the day, where he lets the teacher merely specify that it should be "in the most auspicious part of the day, at a favorable moment." Such detail as is given broadly squares up with times recommended for the initiation ceremony of the student of the Vedas (*brahmacārin*) in the *gṛhyasūtras*, as for example, the bright part of the month, and the lunar mansions (*nakṣatra*) of *tiṣya, hasta, śravaṇa*, or *aśvayuj*.[235] Caraka (via the teacher's speech) names the half year between winter and summer solstice as the appropriate time of the year. The very vagueness of Caraka's recommendations lets us assume that the days and times he prescribes are not specific to the medical tradition, and that by mentioning "the most auspicious part of the day" and so on, he is alluding to mainstream customs of his times, or perhaps more specifically to brahmanic customs as laid out in some *gṛhyasūtra* known to him and his contemporaries. The same goes for Suśruta's treatment of the subject in Sū.2.4, which gives an even more abbreviated form: "on an auspicious day, at an auspicious part of the day, at an auspicious moment, and on an auspicious lunar constellation." Kaśyapa (Vi.2(?).3) follows Caraka's lead in specifying the right time of year to be the period from the winter solstice to the summer solstice (*udagayana*) and adds that the initiation should be performed on an auspicious day in the lunar mansions of *aśvayuj, rohiṇī*, the lunar mansions that contain the word *uttara*,[236] or indeed any other lunar mansion.

In any case, it should be noted that Caraka's teacher is not making an appointment with the student by describing suitable times for the initiation. Instead, the final choice of date and time for the initiation is left to the student: the ball is in his court, and he must become active to set the next series of events in motion.

The Student's Attire and Appearance

The second set of prescriptions details that the student should have shaved his head, fasted, and bathed: These are all methods of outer and inner purification. The practice of coming to the initiation ceremony with a shaved head is commonly prescribed in the *gṛhyasūtras*.[237] The medical student should also should wear an orange robe (*kāṣāyavastra*) and have scented hands. This prescription of dress differs from those for the *brahmacārin* in the *gṛhyasūtras*, in that the Vedic student had to wear two garments, one for the lower part of the body, which could be made out of a variety of materials such as hemp, flax, cotton, or wool, and one for the upper part, which was made from deer, cow, or goat skin.[238] The lower garment could also be dyed in hues of red or yellow, depending on the student's class: reddish-yellow/orange (*kāṣāya*) for brahmins, madder red (*māñjiṣṭha*) for *kṣatriyas*, and turmeric yellow (*hāridra*) for *vaiśyas*.[239] The orange of the medical student's robe may have been chosen in allusion to the color of the brahmin-student's garment. Orange (as well as other hues of red and yellow) is also the prescribed color of the robes of Buddhist monks,[240] but given the context of the passage, it seems more likely that Caraka is alluding to brahmanic than Buddhist conventions. In any case, the similarities of outfit and appearance end here: the *brahmacārin* receives three crucial items at his initiation: a staff (*daṇḍa*), a girdle (*mekhalā*), and a sacred thread (*yajñopavīta*), which play no role at the medical student's initiation, or at least are not mentioned by Caraka or the other medical authors.

Items for the Ceremony

The items the student is to bring to the initiation ceremony include fire sticks and clarified butter, but also imperishable items such as gold and jewels. These are needed to prepare the sacrificial grounds and for use in the sacrifice. The student is to bring both sticks to enclose the sacrificial fire (*paridhi*) and firewood (*samidh*) to fuel it. Ca.Vi.8.11 lists the types of wood used in the ceremony (which are presumably the ones the student brought): *palāśa* (flame of the forest), *iṅguda* (desert date), *udumbara* (cluster fig tree), and *madhūka* (mahua).[241] With the exception of *madhūka*, these are all types of wood also prescribed in the *gṛhyasūtras* for use in the *brahmacārin*'s initiation ceremony.[242] It should also be pointed out that bringing firewood to a teacher is an act specifically associated with someone asking to be accepted as a student. Firewood as an insignia of the student is, for example, attested in the Atharvaveda (11.7),[243] and Kane (1968–77, 2.273) writes that a number of *upaniṣads* describe how the "would-be student came to the teacher with a *samidh* in his hand and told the teacher that he desired to enter the stage of studenthood and begged to be allowed to be a brahmacārī living with the teacher." Mookerji (1947, xxviii–xxix) explains that fetching fuel for the household fire is one of the accepted student's regular duties in the teacher's house, so that approaching a teacher with fuel in hand signifies a student's readiness to serve the teacher and tend his household fire.

The medical student is also to bring "intelligence-promoting foods." How these are then to be used in the ceremony is not explained further by Caraka. However, the *gṛhyasūtras* offer us two scenarios that may be pertinent. First, some *gṛhyasūtras* prescribe that a meal for brahmins should take place before the ceremonies begin.[244] The second scenario relates to the idea of the promotion of intellect: The Āśvalāyana Gṛhyasūtra (1.22.18–19) describes a *saṃskāra* rite[245] that follows the initiation of the *brahmacārin*. This rite, which should be performed on the fourth day after the initiation, is called *medhājanana*, "generation of intelligence."[246] It does not, however, involve any food, so the link between this rite and Caraka's "intellect-promoting foods" may be tenuous.

The Ceremony

When the student arrives bearing the aforementioned items, it is the teacher's turn to prepare the grounds for the ceremony. This is when the initiation ceremony proper begins:

> Having noticed that he [the student] has come near, he [the physician] should first prepare a square piece of ground measuring four *kiṣku*[247] in an even and pure place sloping eastward or toward the north, smeared with cow-dung, strewn with *kuśa* grass, well-bordered on all sides by the fire-sticks, adorned with the mentioned sandalwood, water vessels, silk, golden objects, gold, silver, jewels, pearls, and coral and decorated with pure foods, fragrances, white flowers, fried grain, and whole mustard seeds.[248]

With the grounds ready and the necessary equipment at hand, the teacher now consecrates the ceremony with a ritual in which he offers oblations to gods and sages. The student follows suit.

> There, having kindled a fire with the firewood of flame of the forest,[249] desert date,[250] cluster fig tree,[251] and mahua,[252] facing east and pure as laid down in the method of study, he should thrice sacrifice honey and sweet clarified butter to the fire, addressing mantras, beginning with "Svāhā," to Brahma, Agni, Dhanvantari, Prajāpati, the Aśvins, Indra, and the sages who composed the manuals. And the pupil should grasp him [on his shoulder]. Having sacrificed, he [the pupil] should follow him [the teacher] around the fire, keeping the fire on his right. Having stepped around it, he should salute the brahmins and pay his respects to the physicians.[253]

This ritual follows the same general pattern as the preliminary fire-ritual (*homa*) of a *brahmacārin*'s initiation: the kindling and consecration of the sacrificial fire, the invocation of divinities (here adapted to the medical context by supplementing the gods with the sages who composed the medical treatises), and the making of offerings to them with the fire as medium amid the recitation of prescribed prayers and mantras.[254] The teacher officiates at this ceremony, although there are also brahmins present, which may mean that Caraka envisages the teacher to be a brahmin.[255]

Suśruta's description in Sū.2.4 of this part of the ceremony is very similar to Caraka's:

> A brahmin should be initiated on an auspicious day,[256] at an auspicious part of the day, at an auspicious moment, and in an auspicious lunar

> constellation,[257] on a square platform measuring four *hasta*[258] in a clean and even space and [facing] a favorable direction that has been smeared with cow-dung and strewn with *kuśa* grass. Having worshiped the gods, the sages, and the physicians with jewels, flowers, parched rice, and grains, he should draw lines [upward][259] and sprinkle [the ground with water].[260] Placing a priest to the right,[261] he should kindle a fire with firewood of the cutch tree,[262] flame of the forest, deodar,[263] and Indian quince,[264] or of the four other trees that contain milky sap (banyan,[265] cluster tree, peepul,[266] and mahua), anointed with buttermilk, honey, and clarified butter. He should offer a libation of clarified butter with a ladle, [repeating] the sacred syllable "oṃ," and the formula "bhūr bhuvaḥ svaḥ" according to the rule of the "oblation made with a ladle" [*darvihoma*]. Then, he should hail each deity and the sages with the utterance of "svāhā," and he should let the brahmin student[267] who is to be initiated do the same.

While Caraka's description lets us guess that he is speaking about a brahmin's initiation into medical studies, Suśruta states outright that the ritual he describes is meant for brahmin students. Suśruta's commentator Ḍalhaṇa, however, seems to understand the sole mention of the brahmin student to be indicative of his preeminence among the classes[268] rather than of the ceremony being exclusive to brahmins. Ḍalhaṇa also makes note of a variant reading for *upanayanīyaṃ tu brāhmaṇaṃ*: *upanayanīyas tu brāhmaṇaḥ*, with *upanayanīyas* in an active sense, so that it would mean "the brahmin performing the initiation" (should offer oblations etc.). The student (*śiṣya*) would then be uncategorized in regard to his class. This makes sense, since the next *sūtra* (Su.Sū.2.5) gives clear prescriptions on who can be initiated (namely students of all classes, including *śūdras*).

Suśruta uses very similar wording in his instructions about auspicious times and appropriate preliminary rites (in particular the worship of fire, brahmins and physicians) in Su.Sū.5.7, which describes the right way to go about surgery.

Kaśyapa's description of the initiation ceremony in Vi.2(?).3 is remarkable for its use of expert terminology to list the steps taken to prepare the sacrificial grounds:[269]

> When a student who is desirous of knowledge and endowed with the qualities of a student has approached him, the teacher should initiate [him] in the prescribed way in the half year from the winter to the summer solstice, on an auspicious day in the lunar mansion of *aśvayuj*,

> or *rohiṇī*, in the lunar mansions that contain the word *uttara*,[270] or in another one. Having besmeared a platform the size of a cow hide[271] with cow-dung and water in an auspicious place that slopes east-or northward, and having performed a fire oblation as prescribed, by marking [the ground] with lines, bringing the fire, sweeping the ground [around the fire], and sprinkling [it with water], bringing the sacred *praṇīta*-waters forward, spreading [a layer of grass], straining clarified butter, and offering oblations of clarified butter [to the fire],[272] he sacrifices logs of flame of the forest dipped in clarified butter, calling out: "Hail to Agni, hail to Soma, hail to Prajāpati, hail to Kaśyapa, hail to the two Aśvins, hail to Indra, hail to Dhanvantari, hail to Sarasvatī, hail to Pūrṇabhaga, hail to the well-worshiped Agni!" Having worshiped the brahmin and satisfied him with boiled rice as a donation, and the gods with oblations, and having given the teacher a cup full of water as his fee, he should [say] "To *dadhikrāvan*!"[273] and eat sour milk with his face turned to the east. Having sipped the water, he should circumambulate [the fire], keeping it to his right, and, having touched the teacher's arm, he should say: "I am this son," and, having touched [the teacher's] feet, he should say: "I am this student." (3)

Kaśyapa's account of the ceremony ends with the student's emphatic statements: the student is now initiated, and his studies can commence. This is different from Caraka's (and Suśruta's) treatment of the ceremony, which conclude only after the teacher has instructed the student on his duties as a student and as a practitioner of medicine. Kaśyapa does provide instructions to the disciple regarding his behavior toward the teacher during his apprenticeship in Vi.2(?).6, which could be understood to be part of the ceremony, with *sūtras* 4 and 5 (on the qualities of student and teacher, respectively) as excursions.[274] However, Kaśyapa records no concluding vow by the student, as Caraka does, that would allow us to conclusively define *sūtra* 6 as part of the ceremony.

The Teacher's Speech and the Student's Vow

In Caraka's account of the medical student's initiation, the teacher begins to instruct the student on his duties as a student and as a physician after the ceremonial acts of the fire ritual. This begins in Ca.Vi.8.13 and concludes in 8.14. Menon and Haberman (1970) divide this passage into eight segments: (1) a religious oath, (2) asceticism in the life of a student, (3) the student-teacher relationship, (4) the dedicated physician, (5) the protocol of conduct, (6) the physician's right and obligation to deny his services, (7) postgraduate education, and (8) the successful physician. Menon and Haberman's discussion comprises Ca.Vi.8.13—14 (though only part of 14, i.e., up to the student's avowal to abide by the teacher's rules).[275] Preisendanz (2007, 660–662) suggests a division of the same passage (which she more fittingly entitles "initiatory speech of the master") into four main segments: (1) the student's behavior as student, (2) the student's behavior as a practitioner (already during the period of apprenticeship?),[276] (3) supplementary study, and (4) an admonition regarding correct behavior toward the gods and other figures worthy of respect.[277] The student's assent to the teacher's rules is not categorized as part of the initiatory speech here, but as a division of its own. With Preisendanz's careful analysis in mind, I would like to suggest a more simplified categorization for the purpose of discussing the passage's contents, dividing it into two main topical groups: (1) instructions regarding the student's behavior as a student, and (2) instructions regarding the student's (future) behavior as a practitioner. The second group includes the section Preisendanz entitles "Supplementary Study."

The beginning of Vi.8.13 (i.e., the words "Then, in the presence of a fire, brahmins, and physicians, the teacher should instruct the pupil."), and the second part of Vi.8.14 (i.e., Preisendanz's section 4, "admonition regarding correct behavior toward the Gods" etc., and "assent of the student to act and behave as told") serve as a framework within which the teacher's instructions are contained. This will be discussed separately.

Instructions Regarding the Student's Behaviour as a Student

Caraka's version of these instructions pertain first to the student's appearance and his behavior as a student in general, and second to his behavior toward his teacher in particular:

> Then, in the presence of a fire, brahmins, and physicians, the teacher should instruct the pupil. "You should lead the austere life of a student, wearing a beard, speaking the truth, not eating meat, and having pure pursuits. You should be unselfish, and you should not hold weapons. You must do as I say, unless it [pertains to something that is] hated by the king, life-threatening, greatly unethical, or nonsensical. You should entrust yourself to me, put me first, be obedient to me, and always comply with what is agreeable and beneficial to me. You should live with me attending as a son, a servant, and a supplicant." [278]

The student's appearance and general behavior. These are defined by the instruction that he should lead the life of a *brahmacārin*, which implies a very simple lifestyle that does not allow for finery in dress, or even particular attention to personal hygiene. Though Caraka only concretely mentions wearing a beard and not carrying weapons, it is likely that he is alluding to some other authority prescribing rules for a *brahmacārin*'s lifestyle for further reference, as in his description of the fire ritual. Caraka's specifications that he should always speak the truth, not eat meat, not be selfish, and follow pure pursuits are all general instructions that align well with instructions for the *brahmacārin* found in the *gṛhyasūtras*. Compare, for example, the general rules of conduct for the *brahmacārin* in Āpastamba Gṛhyasūtra 1.3: "He shall be gentle, calm, controlled, modest, firmly resolute, energetic, not given to anger, and free from envy."[279] The general rules for the student in Gautama's Dharmasūtra include not eating meat and a long list of uncouth behaviors that the student must abandon (in favor of pure pursuits).[280] Manu (2.178–180) also warns against eating meat and lying, among a long list of other things.[281] And Baudhāyana Dharmasūtra prescribes that a student "shall speak the truth and remain modest and free from pride."[282]

The medical student's behavior toward his teacher. A student's relationship with his teacher is characterized by his submissiveness, obedience, and devotion to the teacher. His own needs and will are effaced and supplanted instead with those of the teacher. At the same time, the student's submission of will is not absolute. He can, and indeed is required to, disobey the teacher in a number of scenarios: if the teacher asks him to do something disapproved of by the king (i.e., presumably against the law), or to do something life-threatening (perhaps an overly risky, or intentionally lethal medical procedure? Or an action that would threaten the student's life?), to do anything that would be considered greatly unethical (which begs the question whether something "somewhat unethical" would not provide grounds for refusal), or, finally, to do something that makes no sense (i.e., to run pointless errands? Or perhaps to undertake useless treatments?). This list leaves a great many questions open, and again, it seems that Caraka is alluding to case scenarios that were either commonly understood in his times (and thus would have been clear to the student) or otherwise were discussed in more detail elsewhere.[283]

The student's required subservience to the teacher, which could easily take the form of exploitation, is counterbalanced by the close, perhaps even loving nature of their relationship. The student should live with the teacher not just as a servant and a supplicant but also as a son. This implies love, trust, and even a certain amount of rights. Note, however, that the teacher is not explicitly called on to treat the student as his son, though Caraka does write in Vi.8.14 that the teacher "joins himself to the pupil," which suggests that their commitment is mutual. Suśruta goes further than Caraka in spelling out the teacher's obligations to the student in Su.Sū.2.7. According to this passage, a teacher's behavior must mirror the good behavior of the student, or he "would be participating in sin and would become one whose knowledge is fruitless." It is worth noting that though Caraka's student is to live with the teacher as a "servant and a supplicant," none of his actual tasks in the teacher's household are detailed. By comparison, a Veda student's duties are described in detail in many of the *gṛhyasūtras* and *dharmasūtras*. They would typically include fetching firewood (the *samidh* mentioned in the context of the fire ritual) and maintaining the household fire. Another important part of the Veda student's duties would be begging for food (*bhikṣā*). Unsurprisingly, many of the Veda student's principal duties center on performing or taking part in household rituals, and so on. However, we also find more general duties outlined for the Veda student in the ritual textbooks. Kane (1968–77, 2.332), paraphrasing Baudhāyana Dharmasūtra (1.2.34 and 37), writes that a student "should be diligent in doing work that would be pleasing and beneficial to the teacher," which corresponds closely with Caraka's words in Vi.8.13. This resemblance may not be enough to make a case for a direct link between the duties of medical student to his teacher and the rules prescribed for Veda students. However, it also seems unlikely that the similarities are coincidental.

In the *Suśrutasaṃhitā*, we find a similar depiction of the initiation ceremony, with an initiation speech that follows the pattern of the above (though omitting what follows in the *Carakasaṃhitā*, instructions regarding the medical student's behavior as a practitioner) in first outlining what outer appearance and general behavior was required of the student and then defining his duties toward his teacher:

> Then, having lead the pupil three times around the fire, he should say to him with the fire as witness: "Having abandoned passion, anger, avarice, arrogance, conceit, envy, harshness, slander, untruth, laziness, and dishonor, you must have short nails and hair, be clean, wear orange clothing, and by all means be totally devoted to truth, religious observance, celibacy, and respectful salutation. Standing, walking, lying down, sitting, eating, and studying as permitted by me, you should do what is pleasant and wholesome to me. Your behaving otherwise is unrighteous, and the knowledge unproductive, and you will not attain renown.[284]

Suśruta's specifications regarding the student's outer appearance are brief, only detailing that his nails and hair should be short, that he should be clean, and that he should wear orange clothes. On the other hand, his stipulations regarding the student's general behavior are more complex than Caraka's.[285] Suśruta starts off with a long list of negative traits or attitudes the student must give up or avoid and then gives some general directions on good conduct that are decisively brahmanic in tone and evoke the *brahmacārin's* rules of conduct: being devoted to religious observances (*vrata*),[286] celibacy (*brahmacārya*),[287] and salutations (*abhivādana*).[288]

Suśruta's rules regarding a medical student's behavior to the teacher all pertain to the student's obedience to the teacher and demand that the student do nothing without the teacher's permission. Suśruta does not mention that the student lives with the teacher, or that he does service for the teacher, as Caraka does, though both are implied by the demand for complete submission to the teacher's permission.

While Caraka ends his teacher's speech with the statement that a student who does not follow the rules as laid out in the speech should not be taught (Ca.Vi.8.14), Suśruta leaves the moral choice, as it were, with the student who is merely told that not following the rules would be unrighteous and would render his studies fruitless.

Kaśyapa gives the student instructions on what behavior is expected of him during his apprenticeship in Vimānasthāna 2(?).6. Kaśyapa lists a number of positive traits the student should display, as well as some negative ones he shouldn't, and then turns more specifically to the student's relationship with the teacher. A student should be open and trusting toward the teacher and also be emotionally closely attached, feeling for and with the teacher. The student is also reminded that he is not to practice medicine without having been permitted to do so by the teacher first, which signals that his knowledge is sufficient for practice.

The *Aṣṭāṅgasaṃgraha* also offers a short passage on the student's conduct in Sū.2.6–7a, which gives some examples of the student's duties to the teacher. However, this is not part of an initiation speech (Vāgbhaṭa does not describe the initiation ceremony at all) and the student is described in the third person rather than addressed directly in the second person:

> Wearing inferior and different clothes [to the teacher], he should attend upon the teacher as upon a king. He should lie down to sleep only once [the teacher] has lain down to sleep, and he should get up before he does. He should not address him merely by his name, and he should not mimic what is bad.

The student's inferior status and deference to the teacher is visually expressed by his inferior dress. The instruction that he should not go to bed before his teacher and that he must get up first in the morning is also found in rules for the Vedic student in the *dharmasūtras*,[289] as is the instruction regarding respectful address to the teacher.[290] It is not entirely clear to me whether the point about mimicking relates to the teacher's actions or to someone else's. If the former is the case, then there are parallels in the *dharmasūtras* again, which prohibit imitating "the teacher's gait, manners, or speech."[291]

Instructions Regarding the Student's (Future) Behavior as a Practitioner

Caraka is the only one of the medical authors just cited who includes instructions on how to behave as a medical practitioner in the teacher's inauguration speech.[292] Here is the longer part of the teacher's speech, and the most interesting part, in terms of the professional ethics and etiquette it expresses:

> Having been permitted to leave, you should roam around [practicing medicine][293] humbly, attentively, with a focused mind, and modestly, doing whatever needs to be attended to and without envy. Before you leave by permission, you should make an effort to the best of your power to provide the teacher's due.
>
> As a physician who wishes to succeed in practice, to attain wealth, and to gain fame, and who desires heaven after death, you should always, whether you are standing or sitting, wish for the happiness of all living beings, beginning with cows and brahmins. You should strive wholeheartedly for the health of patients. You must not harm patients, even for the sake of living. You should not approach other's wives even in thought, nor any of another's property.
>
> Your clothing and equipment should be modest. You should abstain from alcohol, be virtuous, and have virtuous companions. You should speak gently, purely, justly, joyfully, in a wholesome manner, truthfully, affectionately, and moderately. You should act according to place and time, be mindful, and always strive for perfection in knowledge, diligence, and equipment.
>
> And you should never supply those with medicine who are hated by the king or hostile to the king, hated by eminent persons, or else hostile to eminent persons. And likewise you should not supply all those with medicine who are extremely deformed, evil, and have unpleasant [*duḥkha*] habits, customs, and conduct, those who do not oppose

slander, and those who are about to die. Similarly, [you should not treat] women whose husbands are not present, or who are without guardian.

Also, you should never accept food given by women without permission from their husband or their guardian. And you should enter the patient's home in the right manner by entering together with someone who is known and welcome. You should be well-dressed, your head lowered, and mindful, behaving calmly and with a mind constantly observing everything. And, having entered, your speech, mind, intellect, and senses should be turned to nothing other than the patient, to what is helpful and useful to the patient, or to other conditions the patient has. And you should not disclose any information from the patient's home outside [his home]. And even if you know that the life span of the diseased is diminished, you should not disclose this in a situation in which by speaking [about it], you would harm the diseased or another. Even if you are knowledgeable, you should not boast of your own knowledge too much. Many shrink from one who boasts excessively, even if he is accomplished. (13)

The limits of Ayurveda are indeed not easily passed. Therefore, a diligent person should always keep in constant practice. And this needs to be done like this. Moreover, you should learn excellent conduct ungrudgingly even from adversaries. The whole world is the teacher of the intelligent, and the enemy of fools. Therefore, having considered this, an intelligent person should listen to and follow common advice promoting wealth, fame, restraint, and longevity, even if it is given by an enemy.

Then, afterward, he should say this: "You should always behave properly toward the gods, fire, brahmins, your preceptor, your elders, accomplished ones, and teachers. This fire, all fragrances, flavors, jewels and grains, and the gods as mentioned should prove favorable for you if you conduct yourself properly toward them, and unfavorable, if you behave otherwise." When the teacher has said that, the pupil should answer "So be it." If he acts according to these instructions, he should be taught; otherwise, however, he should not be taught. And a teacher who teaches a suitable pupil obtains the said fruits of teaching and other unmentioned qualities that bring prosperity, and he joins himself to the pupil. Thus the rule for teaching has been stated. (14)[294]

According to this speech, then, the medical student's studies are completed when he has received permission by his teacher to go forth to practice medicine on his own. Before he can leave, however, he is admonished to make efforts to give the teacher his due. There is no clarification on what this fee consists of—money, or goods, or services. It may not have been a set amount in any case. The words "you should strive to the best of your power" imply that the teacher may have been flexible in his demands, asking only for what he (or perhaps even the student) thought was within the limits of what the student could afford. Once he has settled his debt to the teacher, the student is to "roam around [practicing medicine]"—to practice medicine as an itinerant physician rather than as one with a practice in a settled location. From this moment on, he needs to follow certain rules concerning his personal and professional behavior. The teacher gives detailed advice on how "to succeed in practice, to attain wealth, and to gain fame." This advice concerns the physician's attitudes, his appearance, his general conduct and manners, and finally his relationships with patients and how to interact with them. Advice on his attitude represents the physician's ethics—the moral motivations for his actions; the rest of the teacher's advice pertains to etiquette: the rules that govern a physician's social and professional behavior. These may reflect the conventional cultural norms of Caraka's times, but may also reflect an underlying ethic that is more specific to the medical world.

As noted, Caraka alone among the medical authors places advice on a physician's conduct within the initiation speech. The position of this advice is somewhat incongruous, given its context—the initiation. Since the initiation precedes the commencement of studies, this advice comes at a time long before the student will practice on his own. It would seem that advice on how to practice medicine would make rather more sense at the end of the student's apprenticeship, when he is about to embark on his own independent practice. However, while the advice does seem to refer to the time when a student has been released from his apprenticeship (as indicated by the preceding "Having been permitted to leave, you should roam around [practicing medicine]"), it is also possible that it refers to the period of the student's apprenticeship as well.[295] It seems likely, for example, that a student would accompany his teacher on his rounds as part of learning the trade, in which case advice on how to behave in a patient's house would be crucial.

The ethical attitudes described in the teacher's speech encompass philanthropy, but also a wider concern for the happiness of all living beings. They also include commitment to preserving or establishing the patient's welfare. Wishing happiness for all beings is well known as part of Buddhist thought,[296] but Caraka's specification that wishing all beings well should begin with cows and brahmins places this notion squarely into a brahmanic context.

The passage beginning "The limits of Ayurveda are indeed not easily passed" describes the necessity of continuing study and constant practice in order to maintain and perfect one's knowledge and skill as a physician. This is already touched on some paragraphs earlier, where the student is told that he should "always strive for perfection in knowledge, diligence, and equipment." Continuing learning is, however, not confined to medical knowledge but includes any advice on how to conduct oneself properly. Knowledge can be derived from sources other than the student's teacher: the "whole world is the teacher of the intelligent," and good advice can even be obtained from one's enemies. This constitutes a lesson in humility. The student is confronted with the fact not only that his knowledge can never be complete and must always be worked on but also that he must even seek and accept advice from his adversaries. The importance of gaining knowledge supersedes any considerations of ego and self-importance. This suggests to me that knowledge and skill are part of the physician's ethic: Acquiring, preserving, nurturing, and applying knowledge is as much a moral as a practical requirement of the physician.

The physician's etiquette as outlined in the teacher's speech concerns his general appearance and conduct, whom he should not treat, and his specific behavior in the patient's house. The topic of whom the physician should reject as patient and why he should do so has already been discussed.[297] Caraka's instructions here broadly follow those of Vi.3.45 and Si.2.4–6, and add only two additional cases in which treatment would be deemed improper: a physician must stay away from women whose husbands are not present or who are without guardian. Unlike the other cases, in which treatment is absolutely forbidden, the first scenario describes a temporary situation, which necessitates postponement rather than complete abandonment of treatment. The second may allude to a temporary situation but could also describe women who are permanently without guardian, and thus would be excluded from medical care for good.

Suśruta also gives a list of persons a physician should not treat (and whom he should)[298] in the passage following his version of the initiation ceremony. This does not, however, seem to be part of the initiation ceremony proper,[299] though Suśruta concludes his list with the words "Thus knowledge shines and one attains friends, fame, religious merit, wealth, and pleasure"—similar goals to the ones Caraka's teacher sets in his speech (i.e., success, wealth, fame, and heaven after death). Vāgbhaṭa's treatment of the subject can similarly be found in his chapter on the initiation of the student, in which there is, however, no description of the initiation ceremony itself.[300]

In the teacher's speech in the *Carakasaṃhitā*, not only a physician's general appearance and conduct but also his behavior to his patients are guided by the principles of conformity and modesty. He should be inconspicuous, pleasant, and not threatening in any way. The teacher's description of how to behave in the patient's house is quite detailed and reads like a step-by-step guide to the proper house visit. The first rule is to come to the patient's house accompanied by someone who is known and welcome. This is likely to be the messenger who summoned the physician.[301] The physician's behavior during his visit should be composed and modest. It is imperative for him to observe everything closely so that he can arrive at a diagnosis. He should be extremely attentive to the patient's needs and to his care, and not let himself get distracted by other occurrences in the household. He must respect the confidentiality of anything he witnesses during his visit to the patient's home, and this discretion includes not only information about the patient's condition but also any other information regarding the patient's home. The physician must generally take care with how to deal with information on the patient's condition: If a patient's condition is fatal and his death near, he may not divulge this information to the patient himself if he judges that informing him will cause damage to the patient, or to his relatives.[302] Finally, the teacher turns again to the physician's self-representation, and warns him not to boast of his knowledge and achievements, since this cannot but alienate his patients.

The emphasis on modesty in attire and bearing that characterizes the model physician in this speech may reflect his uneasy status in society. He is a figure of authority whom patients trust and respect and whose services they depend on. But at the same time he is someone who practices a trade, moreover one that has connotations of impurity. Then again, he is educated and powerful with his specialized knowledge, which makes the hierarchy less clear. In any case, the physician must make sure his patients' needs are met, and this includes making them comfortable with his presence. Adhering to confidentiality, for example, is very much part of this policy of posing no threat and being agreeable to the patient. Patients may resent their very need of the physician, and may fear his power over them, and he must assuage these fears. In short, a physician must tread carefully. By behaving in certain ways, he is creating a public image of himself that allows him to fit into society and to be accepted by his patients. This is as much the key to his success as his medical knowledge and skill. The professional skills of a doctor must therefore include an understanding of social circumstances and an aptitude to adapt to them. In this part of the speech, then, the teacher is revealing an essential part of medical practice. He is providing the medical man's equivalent of Dale Carnegie's guidance in *How to Win Friends and Influence People.*

Perhaps not all of it must necessarily be understood in the light of pleasing clients to secure their custom. While the rules of conduct may be partly aimed at the utilitarian goal of making a living, one could certainly also make the argument that the prescriptions may pertain to an external manifestation of an internalized, deontological ethic. Modesty in dress and behavior can reflect true freedom from vanity and arrogance. The physician may cultivate a real sense of responsibility for the patient's welfare that does not spring from self-interest, but from a sense of duty and the rights of others. In any case, self-interest and a sense of duty need not be mutually exclusive, since they can be directed at the same ultimate, or intermediate goal (in this case, the welfare of the patient). On the other hand, postulating a deontological ethic may be reading rather too much between the lines. The teacher, after all, says quite clearly that all of his instructions must be followed if a physician wishes for success, wealth, and so on. In other words, he does not advocate doing good for its own sake. The speech also reflects an epistemology in which there is a predictable order to life. Certain actions bring about certain effects—if you do A, B must follow. The benefits of wealth, fame, heaven after death, and so on that a physician reaps from his good works are not only his just but also his expected reward.

One further important point needs to be made: Many of the instructions regarding the physician's conduct can be found in another context, for example in the section on good conduct in Ca.Sū.8.18–33. These long and detailed prescriptions pertain to everyone, and whoever follows the rules of good conduct not only lives a long life free from disease but also "fills the human world with fame, is highly thought of by good persons, [and] acquires virtue and wealth, and the friendship of all beings."[303] Here we find admonitions such as one should not disclose secrets, one should not be conceited, one should be skilled and competent and not envious.[304] The section on good conduct begins with the instruction that one should honor gods, cows, brahmins, preceptors, the elders, accomplished persons, and teachers.[305] This corresponds closely with the last admonition the teacher gives at the end of his speech at the medical student's initiation. ("You should always behave properly toward the gods, fire, brahmins, your preceptor, your elders, accomplished ones, and teachers.") Further comparison confirms that what Caraka envisions as a physician's good conduct does not really differ from what he recommends for everyone else. The specifications concerning a physician's conduct in the teacher's speech function as a condensation of the more detailed rules of general good conduct in Ca.Sū.8. The physician's code of conduct reiterates the essence of what good conduct should be, leaving aside such rules as have no bearing on the specific situation of a physician.

The teacher's final admonition (that the student should always honor the gods, fire, brahmins, etc.) seems in some ways the most significant part of the speech, since it alone is linked with the fire ritual and the ceremonial items by the teacher's statement "this fire, all fragrances, flavors, jewels and grains, and the gods as mentioned should prove favorable for you if you conduct yourself properly toward them, and unfavorable, if you behave otherwise." As noted, the prescription to honor the gods and so on is not specific to a physician's education or his medical practice but rather relates to the wider issue of the correct conduct of an adult. The ceremony concludes with the student agreeing to abide by the rules set out in the speech. Caraka adds that a teacher should only teach a student who adheres to these rules, and that the teacher himself will be rewarded with the fruits of teaching, which include wealth. Suśruta, by contrast, does not describe the student's vow to abide by the rules set out by the teacher but rather lets the teacher conclude his speech with his own vow that he must behave in a proper manner toward the student, describing the negative consequences for himself if he does not do his duty to the student.[306]

The Suśrutasaṃhitā on physicians' professional conduct. While Suśruta does not place the subject of the new physician's professional conduct within the context of the medical student's initiation, his treatment of the subject is very similar to that described in the *Carakasaṃhitā*. Suśruta devotes an entire (albeit short) chapter to the physician's entry into the profession, which covers advice not only on how to behave as a physician but also, as noted, on whom a physician should or should not treat. A physician's etiquette is described in Su.Sū.10.3 and 9:

> "A physician who sets out on this path should have understood the system, and have practiced the goals of the system. He should have witnessed operations, and developed practical experience and be involved in discussing the discipline. He must be licensed by the king. He should be clean, keep his nails and hair short, and dress in a white garment. He should have an umbrella, carry a stick, wear sandals, and have a modest outfit. He should be cheerful, well-spoken, and honest. He should be a friend to all creatures and keep good company." (3)

> *"One should not sit in the same place as the women, nor live with them, or joke with them. The best physicians should not accept anything given to them by the women, except food.* (9)"[307]

Again, we find the emphasis on knowledge and and practical skills. Suśruta also gives some attention to the physician's outer appearance as well as to his character, both of which conform with Caraka's prescriptions. The attributes that describe a physician's character—cheerfulness, honesty, and being a friend to all creatures—go beyond mere etiquette. They describe someone who is kind and good in a moral sense.

The sentences in between (i.e., 4–8) that are not given here concern the method of diagnosis, and who is difficult to treat.

The concluding verse, presented by Suśruta as a quote, refers to physicians' behavior toward women. Taken out of its context, the verse seems to refer not only to female patients, or females connected to patients, but to women in general. The word translated "to live with them," *saṃvāsa*, may also be rendered "to associate [with]" or even "to have a sexual connection [with]." It seems unlikely (though not impossible) that the verse is generally advocating a celibate life, or that one live separately from women (i.e., not to marry). In keeping with parallel prescriptions from the *Carakasaṃhitā* and the *Kāśyapasaṃhitā*, it seems more likely that the verse refers to physicians' visits to a patient's home, where they should not associate with the women in the house.

Suśruta devotes chapter 24 of the Cikitsāsthāna to the topic of the healthy regimen, of which general good conduct (*sadvṛtta*) is a subsection. In particular, the content of Cik.24.89 and 90 is very similar to what Suśruta has to say on good professional conduct. The similarities concern outer appearance (cleanliness, having short nails and hair, wearing white clothes, holding an umbrella and a stick) but also include being accompanied by a good companion or assistant. In a statement reminiscent of Caraka's "Having been permitted to go" in Ca.Vi.8.13, Suśruta also notes that one should only go forth with the permission of one's preceptor and the elders,[308] and further includes a list of persons with whom not to consort, which again is similar to Caraka's list in Ca.Vi.8.13 of whom not to supply with medicine. It seems to me that Su.Cik.24.89–90, with its similarities to Su.Sū.10. and to Ca.Vi.8.13, may be describing professional rather than general good conduct, that is, that this section may be displaced. Su.Cik.24.89, though a non sequitur to the preceding sentence, begins with *tatrādita eva*, "In regard to this, from the very beginning," which would fit in nicely with the scenario of a physician commencing his medical practice. On the other hand, the noted advice concerning personal hygiene and apparel occur in all sections on general good conduct in the medical treatises, and thus do seem to refer to common etiquette.

The Kāśyapasaṃhitā on physicians' professional conduct. Kaśyapa deals with the rules of conduct for physicians in Vimānasthāna 2(?).8, after rules concerning the correct way of studying.[309] His treatment of the subject follows Caraka's quite closely:

> Having finished his studies, and having been permitted to go, he should go forth, wearing white clothes, with his hair tied together, calm, looking toward the ground, speaking first, and bright-faced. He should not enter the patient's house without having been summoned, and on entering he should consider the omens. He should not observe anything but the patient. And he ought neither to joke around with the women in the patient's household, even if they are servants, and he certainly ought not accept irreverence or disrespect from them. He must address them by their title of respect, and must not behave overly affectionately with them. Also, he should not take anything from women without the knowledge of their husband. He should not enter unknown. He should not speak or sit with a woman in private, and he should not look at her or laugh at her when she is naked. He should ignore her if she is affectionate, and should not reveal [this]. He must not disclose any secret from the patient's household to the public, and he must not gossip about problems in the patient's household.
>
> If he has seen signs of [the patient's] impending death, he should not tell the patient the truth. He should always comfort [him]. He should never approach someone whose body is overpowered by Death, who has an incurable disease, or who has no equipment. He should not prescribe medicine in the wrong order, and he should not make it dependent on another.[310] He should not use medicine made by himself. He should know about the altered states of the body, medicine, disease, and age.
>
> He should always have stores of incense, collyrium, and medicines. He should not quarrel with other physicians, and he should prepare medicine together with them. Confident and fearless if the occasion arises, he should always speak very clearly, entertainingly, gently, with arguments by analogy,[311] persuasively, consistently, and virtuously. A physician who wishes all beings well is happy in both this and the other world.

As we can see, Kaśyapa offers more or less the same advice as Caraka and Suśruta, though with a much greater emphasis on taking care when associating with women. His advice concerning communications with colleagues stands out, since neither Caraka nor Suśruta make mention of contact with other doctors in the quoted passages.[312] Kaśyapa prescribes peaceful interactions between colleagues that may even include preparing medicines together. The guidance Kaśyapa gives on interaction between professionals (i.e., that physicians should not compete with their colleagues and should prepare medicines together with them) is unique and finds no parallel in the other medical treatises.

There is no chapter on good conduct in the version of the *Kāśyapasaṃhitā* that is available to us to compare with this section on professional conduct.

The Aṣṭāṅgasaṃgraha on physicians' professional conduct. Vāgbhaṭa's description of a physician's professional conduct in the *Aṣṭāṅgasaṃgraha* (Sū.2.7–20) is part of the chapter "*śiṣyopanayanīya,*" "Initiation of the Student." Preceded by the topics of how to choose a student, how to undertake study, and what a student's proper behavior is, and followed by Vāgbhaṭa's version of the four pillars of treatment, this section addresses the same points as Caraka does in Ca.Vi.8.13, with further parallels to Ca.Sū.9 (Caraka's section on the four pillars) and Su.Sū.3. There is some overlap concerning physical appearance and attire (cleanliness, wearing shoes, holding an umbrella, etc.) with Vāgbhaṭa's chapter on daily regimen (*dinacaryā*) in Sūtrasthāna 3 (and particularly As.Sū.3.41–42), but only few parallels beyond that:

> One who is irrefutable, unopposed, firm, and friendly, and has nice looks, who has studied widely, knows the appropriate time [for any activity], has mastered the treatise and knows the *Arthaśāstra,*[313] who attends to those without guardian when they are ill, as if they were his own sons, and who has been authorized by his teacher deserves the title "physician." (7cd–9ab) One who knows only the discipline's theory but is not completely skilled in medical practice becomes confused on meeting a patient, like a coward on reaching a battle. (9cd–10ab) However, one who performs medical practice leaving out the discipline's theory out of boldness is despised by respectable people and meets with punishment by the king. (10cd–11ab) One who has the fourfold knowledge of cause, symptom, cure, and prevention of diseases is the best physician and fit for a king. (11cd–12ab) A weapon, learning, and water depend on their recipient to manifest their merits and defects; therefore, one should further one's knowledge with erudition. (12cd–13ab) Learning is the light, one's wide intellect is the perception; a physician who undertakes treatment with both harmoniously joined cannot do wrong. (13cd–14ab) A physician who visits [his patients] only after he has been called, who is well-dressed, sets out at auspicious moments, pays attention to the patient's concerns only, not to anything else, examines diseases properly according to their characteristics, such as causes, and so on, does not spread any embarrassing[314] rumours about him

> [i.e., the patient] outside [his home], and knows how to treat [a disease] quickly, not losing time for its treatment, attains success. (14cd–17ab) He should not accept a gift given by women in the absence of their guardian, and he should avoid having secrets or joking with them. (17cd–18ab) A physician [should avoid] patients who are despised by the king, by respectable persons, and by physicians, who are their enemies and hostile, who are violent, afflicted by sorrow, cowardly, and ungrateful and who think themselves physicians, and who are unequipped, inattentive, not compliant, or very old. (18cd–19)[315]

In conclusion, the medical student's initiation ceremony is strikingly similar to that of the Vedic student. At the same time, there are some significant formal differences: the medical student is not invested with the Vedic student's accoutrements of staff, girdle, and sacred thread. He also is not taught the Sāvitrī prayer as part of a first lesson in the ceremony. And the rules of conduct during his apprenticeship that the teacher lays out do not include religious duties, such as performing morning rituals and so on. Neither is the medical student told that he must tend to the household fire or that he must beg in other households for his food—basic duties for the *brahmacārin*. His duties are defined quite simply as submission and obedience to his teacher (which are also important characteristics of the *brahmacārin*), while more attention is given to his general behavior. Apart from these differences, the medical authors' treatment of the subject broadly conforms with that of the authors of the *dharmasūtras*. The similarity to the Vedic student's initiation throws up a number of questions. The first is whether the medical authors' depiction of the initiation ceremony was based on actual ceremonies taking place in their times (i.e., the medical authors were writing as witnesses of such ceremonies). Alternatively, their descriptions could be expressions of what they envisioned or wished to promote as an ideal procedure for the commencement of medical education. I tend to assume that the described initiation ceremonies, or at least ceremonies similar to them, did indeed take place, since they are described in several of the medical treatises, and in particular in both the *Carakasaṃhitā* and the *Suśrutasaṃhitā*. While one author may have taken his cue from another (as in the case of the *Aṣṭāṅgasaṃgraha*, where the use of the *Suśrutasaṃhitā* and the *Carakasaṃhitā* as templates is overtly acknowledged), it seems unlikely that Suśruta or Caraka would paraphrase the other's description of an initiation ceremony not known to him without at least commenting on it, or adding the phrase "some say" (used in other instances to denote that the described procedure was known by hearsay) to it. Assuming then that such initiations took place, the question is still left open as to how the medical student's initiation was positioned vis-à-vis the religious student's initiation (which may be indicative of the wider issue of how the medical profession was positioned, or positioned itself, within brahmanic culture). The religious student's initiation (or at least our textual evidence for it) is older than that of the medical student.[316] It therefore seems likely that the latter is modeled on the former. That the medical treatises display a knowledge of the *brahmacārin*'s initiation by referring to the "twice–born" *(dvija)*[317] a number of times,[318] further corroborates the idea that the medical student's initiation follows the pattern of the *brahmacārin*'s initiation. But do the ceremonies share the same significance?

A *brahmacārin*'s initiation makes him fit to study the Vedas. It also confers on him the status of a twice-born, which is significant for his position in society. According to Scharfe (2002, 88), a boy is in some sense a *śūdra* before his initiation,[319] but he joins the upper classes, the *āryas*, afterward.

The medical student's initiation, on the other hand, makes him fit to receive tuition on medicine. According to the medical authors, the medical student's initiation and his subsequent education are also meant to confer on him a heightened status in society. The medical authors agree that a well-educated physician will attain wealth and fame. This positive image from within the medical tradition, however, contrasts with a rather negative one from a brahmanic source: In the authoritative *Manusmṛti*, physicians are grouped among those who are unfit to be invited to divine or ancestral offerings, since what is given to physicians there "turns into pus and blood."[320] Manu declares that a brahmin must never eat food given by a physician (4.212), since "the food of a physician is pus" (4.220). He also defines physicians who act crookedly as "thorns" to society (9.259), though this should not refer to honest physicians.[321]

And yet, despite this rather negative imagery from a brahmanic source, the medical authors seem to position themselves and the medical community they represent within the mainstream of brahmanic society, even claiming a position in its higher ranks. There are several possible explanations for this seeming paradox. One is that the negative image of the physician in the *Manusmṛti* was not representative of the actual status physicians held in society. In this case, the medical authors' self-representation may simply be a reflection of reality. Another explanation is that physicians held a difficult position in society in which they were not fully accepted by the higher circles. In that case, their appropriation of brahmanic customs, and particularly their introducing formal procedures of education and standards of practice, may have represented a concerted effort to establish their craft as a respectable profession and themselves as deserving of esteem. This explanation jars a bit, since it seems unlikely that a group (i.e., brahmins) that makes a claim of superiority to others and is by its nature exclusive should welcome an appropriation of its rites and customs as a tactic to climb into its ranks. It makes more sense the other way around: brahmins appropriated medical knowledge from outside their own tradition, introducing elements from their culture into it. This would account for the fact that members of the higher classes—those with access to brahmanic customs—became physicians themselves, though it does not solve the problem of the negative representation of physicians in orthodox brahmanic literature.[322]

With all its similarities of form and function, we must ask whether the medical student's initiation was meant to complement or even to replace the Vedic ritual. While this is not stated overtly anywhere in the medical treatises, an interesting passage from the *Carakasaṃhitā* shows that the possibility of medical education superseding religious education may have been considered:

> "Everyone admires a twice-born[323] physician who is courteous, wise, self-disciplined, and a master of his subject. He is like a guru, a master of life itself. On completing his studentship a physician is said to be born again: the title 'doctor' [Skt. *vaidya*] is earned, not inherited. On completing his studentship, a spirit, be it divine or heroic, enters firmly into him because of his knowledge: that is why the physician is called 'twice-born.'"[324]

Here, then, the second birth does not happen through the initiation into Vedic studies, but through the completion of (note: not the initiation into) medical studies. Interestingly, there is a variant reading of this passage, in which all mention of "twice–born" and so on is replaced with terms for "thrice-born" and so on.[325] Reading "thrice-born" would mean that the third birth on completing medical studies would follow the second birth of the initiation into Vedic studies—that medical studies do not stand in place of religious studies but follow and complement them. At the same time, a third birth may be interpreted as placing the "thrice-born" into a more exalted position than the merely "twice-born." Caraka, however, does not discuss the implications of this passage (nor does Cakrapāṇidatta). Let us remember, though, that Caraka, when describing how to identify a suitable student, recommends that he should come from a family of physicians (or that he should behave as such) but does not comment on which stratum of society the student should come from otherwise.[326] The connection to the medical world is apparently of more importance to Caraka than distinctions of class. This contrasts with Suśruta's class-based dictum that a physician should initiate a brahmin, *kṣatriya*, or *vaiśya* from a good family, or even a *śūdra*.[327]

Leaving aside considerations concerning class, or the relation of the procedures proposed by the medical authors to those known from legal and religious literature, the use of formal procedures delineating the rules and guidelines of education and the credo of the profession generally serves the purpose of reassuring the public (of whatever class) of the trustworthiness of the expert group adhering to them. This is significant for an expert group that makes its living from its specialist knowledge. The first part of Caraka's teacher's speech lays out an established and accepted pattern of teacher–pupil interaction, thus presenting medical education as part of an orthodoxy. The second part of the speech, which gives details on how a physician is to act professionally, is perhaps even more relevant to how the public perceived physicians. This perception would have been subject to both the public knowing that physicians had a set of rules of professional conduct and to the public directly experiencing or witnessing the consequences of the rules of conduct: a physician's good behavior.

Caraka's teacher's speech has been dubbed "The medical student's oath," or just "Caraka's Oath," in parallel to the Hippocratic Oath, by some authors.[328] As I have pointed out elsewhere, the passage in Caraka's text is not actually conceived as an oath, but as an exposition on the correct method of teaching.[329] However, the student is to agree with the teacher's demands at the end of the speech (Ca.Vi.8.14) and thus can be understood to pledge to uphold the rules set out by the teacher, that is, to swear an oath. Note that the student's assent to the teacher's rules is a prerequisite to his being taken up as an apprentice, not to his taking up work as a physician. At the same time, his promise is not limited to the period of his apprenticeship, so his assent to the teacher's exposition on correct professional behavior should be binding for the duration of his professional life. The main question is, then, whether the teacher's speech and the student's concluding assent were held publicly and witnessed by others. Vowing privately (or in the presence of the person exacting the vow) to behave in certain ways can be very meaningful to the person undertaking the vow. However, publicly declaring one's intention to uphold certain rules of conduct fulfills a further function: An oath gives the public (and indeed the budding professional himself) information about what a professional group defines as its responsibilities, and what behavior it deems appropriate. It lets the public know what to expect of a member of a professional group. The student's public pledge to adhere to the stated rules makes him accountable not only to his own conscience but also to those who have heard his vow and know the rules he is meant to follow. This point of contact between professional and public is significant, since the expert group depends on the community for the recognition of its expertise and the grant of professional authority. The dependence of the expert group on the public is why professional norms—publicly stated or not—cannot simply be expressions of the expert group's interests but must fulfill standards that relate to the needs of the larger community, as well as adhering to existing laws.

In the case of the medical student's initiation in the *Carakasaṃhitā*, the teacher's speech and the student's vow do not take place in full public, but certainly in the presence of a number of witnesses: Caraka describes the presence of brahmins and physicians at the beginning of Vi.8.13. The physicians could be understood as representatives of the expert group, and the brahmins as public witnesses to the ceremony (in addition to their role in the performance of the initiation ritual). The involvement of brahmins in the ceremony is interesting in that it points to their accepting and sanctioning the procedures of medical education, and thus in some sense authorizing the practice of medicine. They are also rather high-profile witnesses to the student's vow, which may have been an important factor in ensuring that the medical student keep to his vows beyond the period of his apprenticeship. Caraka does not describe any enforcement of the rules of conduct by an expert group of physicians. Indeed, physicians may not have grouped together to form a coherent professional group at all: We have only few clues about professional interaction between physicians, the presence of physicians at the medical student's initiation being one of them. During the medical student's apprenticeship, his teacher can enforce his good behavior by threatening the withdrawal of tuition. Caraka states as much at the end of Vi.8.14. And there is some idea that, by swearing an oath as part of the ceremony, the student has made himself subject to the powers of the "fire, all fragrances, flavors, jewels and grains, and the gods," which may prove favorable or unfavorable to him depending on his future behavior. This, however, seems to refer only to the preceding "You should always behave properly toward the gods, fire, brahmins, your preceptor, your elders, accomplished ones, and teachers" rather than to the other rules the teacher has laid out. On the other hand, Caraka finally states in the last sentences of Vi.8.14 that a teacher should only teach a student who abides by the stated rules, so that there is a sense that the ceremony was meant to provide a formal framework for a kind of contract between student and teacher.

According to Thomas Oberlies, a number of actions are described as crucial elements in the formal exchange of contracts in brahmanic *dharma* literature: the speaking of (contractual) words, the pouring of water, the reaching of the right hand, the clockwise circumambulation of the fire, the sacrificing into the fire, and finally, the taking of seven steps together.[330] Added to these is another basic feature: that the contract be concluded in front of a fire as witness.[331] In the *Carakasaṃhitā*, not only the fire but also the grains, ornaments, and so on on the sacrificial platform and the gods are summoned as witnesses to the ceremony and in particular to the student's promise to behave well in the future. Caraka's ceremony includes the elements of speaking contractual words (i.e., the teacher's speech and the student's words of assent), the sacrificing into the fire, and the clockwise circumambulation around it. Suśruta and Kaśyapa mention water as part of the ceremony, but not its pouring. None of the medical authors mentions grasping the right hand or taking seven steps together. The latter may be specific to the wedding ceremonies. However, the pouring of water, over hands in particular, seems to have been an important element in oaths.[332] In other words, the medical authors' descriptions of the ceremony fits many, but not all, of the criteria that are found in *dharma* literature as formal elements of concluding a contract.

As a final point of discussion, I would like to reiterate that what Caraka lays out as a physician's good conduct is essentially the same as what he prescribes as good conduct in general, the former being a synopsis of the latter, albeit with some additional detail concerning a physician's interaction with patients. The similarity between general good conduct and good professional conduct is also present in the *Suśrutasaṃhitā*. The *Aṣṭāṅgahṛdayasaṃhitā* gives advice similar to that found in the *Suśrutasaṃhitā* but does not provide a code of conduct for the physician.[333] Conversely, the *Kāśyapasaṃhitā* gives an account of a physician's professional conduct similar to that of Caraka but does not offer any code of conduct for the general public. In the case of the *Aṣṭāṅgasaṃgraha*, there is some overlap between the rules of the daily regimen[334] and the rules of conduct for the physician. These concern physical appearance and attire (cleanliness, wearing shoes and holding an umbrella, etc.). However, there are only few parallels beyond that, though also no contradictions to what is recommended as appropriate behavior for the physician.

The treatises' descriptions of a physician's good professional behaviour are similar enough to each other (albeit with different emphases in each) to warrant the statement that the treatises share a common code of professional ethics. More tentatively, it is also possible to say that this code is linked with a wider ethic of good conduct laid out by the medical authors.

There is also some similarity to what several of the *dharmasūtras* and *gṛhyasūtras* have to say on the proper conduct of a bath-graduate—a *brahmacārin* who has finished his study of the Veda and has bathed to signal the end of his studentship and his entry into the next phase of his life. For example, similar prescriptions for outer appearance (short hair and nails, white or uncolored clothes, holding an umbrella and a stick, etc.) appear in several instances.[335] Śaṅkhāyana Gṛhyasūtra 3.1 describes the occasion of the graduate's bath.[336] Here, he not only takes a bath but has his hair and nails cut, is dressed in new garments and shoes, and is given an umbrella and a stick: the very outfit proposed by the medical authors. This is the bath-graduate's proper attire from now on. In some sense, wearing these clothes may be understood as a reference to the successful completion of studies and to the moment in which the graduation is formally acknowledged by the bath and so on. The modern equivalent would be the use of an honorific title as an outward sign of achievement and a reference to having successfully partaken in a course of study. The medical authors do not describe a formal completion of medical studies other than referring to the teacher's permission to leave. However, the prescription that a physician should wear white clothes, and so on may serve as an oblique reference to the completion of medical studies. The parallels in the *Manusmṛti*, however, go beyond injunctions on outer appearance: Manu.4.133–134[337] speaks of whom not to consort with, and while the list is not an exact match with those of the medical authors, it does include some of the same persons, such as unrighteous persons and other men's wives. Manu (4.138) also admonishes that "he should say what is true, and should say what is pleasant; he should not say what is true but unpleasant, and he should not say what is pleasant but untrue."[338]

In their rules of professional conduct, then, the medical authors again display an affinity—though not a complete correspondence—with brahmanic religious law literature.

3

On Continued Learning and Interaction with Peers

I HAVE SUGGESTED above that knowledge and skill are a key part of the physician's ethic, and that acquiring, preserving, nurturing, and applying knowledge is a moral requirement of the physician. Before a physician can begin his independent practice, he must make sure that he has studied the entire discipline with his teacher. However, once acquired, the attained knowledge must be nurtured and firmed. Therefore, learning and practice are not just confined to the formal period of study under a teacher but form an inextricable part of the physician's professional life.

Caraka states in Vi.8.5 that when a student has "studied the entire discipline by his [the teacher's] gracious aid, he should strive hard in the right manner for a firm grasp of the discipline, an excellent command of its terminology, an understanding of its theories, and for the ability to relate them." Suśruta similarly admonishes in Sū.3.56 that "one who has completed his studies should strive for excellence of speech, an understanding of theory, confidence, dexterity in procedures, repeated practice of them, and success." Suśruta emphasizes that even experts must supplement their knowledge with ideas from other disciplines to arrive at a fuller understanding of their own area of expertise.[339]

Caraka explains that study, teaching, and discussion with experts are the means through which one can retain and deepen one's knowledge.[340] A lesson on how to go about studying follows (already discussed). Although teaching is categorized as a means to attain a firm grasp of the discipline, and so on, what Caraka then describes as the method of teaching (which is essentially presented as a guide on how to choose a student and how to initiate him) does not actually relate to furthering a physician's understanding of the science through the act of teaching. The third means to extending and deepening one's knowledge, that is, discussion with experts, on the other hand, is discussed more pertinently.[341] Caraka begins his long exposition on debate in Vi.8.15 with an explanation on why a physician should take part in debates:

> A physician should engage in discussions with another physician. A discussion with specialists promotes perseverance in and competition[342] for knowledge. Moreover, it develops experience, lends eloquence, and brightens fame.
>
> For one who is uncertain about what was heard (i.e., taught orally) previously, it removes uncertainty in what was heard through hearing it again. And for one who is not uncertain about what has been heard, it produces greater conviction.[343] It even brings some topic that has not been heard before into hearing range. A kind teacher teaches an eager student a subject considered secret gradually, [but] in debate with another, he, wishing to win [the discussion], tells it in compressed form on account of competitiveness.[344] Therefore, the experts recommend holding discussions with specialists.

Debate, then, exposes the participant to new ideas, or to new interpretations of established knowledge. It is meant to reinforce and enhance what he already knows. Interestingly, the idea that his knowledge might be challenged as wrong—and perhaps even rightly so—is not brought up here. The premise seems to be that the physician's knowledge is sound, if incomplete. Caraka's exposition on debate[345] is quite complicated, differentiating between friendly and hostile debate; superior, inferior, and equal debating partners; and even ignorant or knowledgeable audiences, and discussing how to deal with the implications the different constellations of these factors entail.[346] In a friendly discussion with a learned debating partner, Caraka advises that one should not hold on to one's views beyond a reasonable point, which implies that one's previous knowledge was not just incomplete but also wrong. Hostile debate with a learned opponent is not recommended. In all other case scenarios, however, one is meant to defeat one's debating partner by a variety of means.[347] These means are summarized by Dominik Wujastyk as follows:

> One should bamboozle and ridicule the opponent, and deny him the opportunity of speaking. One should use long words to tell him that his proposition does not stand, and one should call to him saying that he needs another year of education or that he has not had a teacher.[348]

In spite of such ruses, the tone in which discussion is conducted is generally meant to remain cordial. Caraka also emphasizes that "a discussion taking place among physicians should be about Ayurveda only and not about anything else."[349] He further admonishes that

> one should make every argument after having thoroughly considered all these, not [saying] what is irrelevant or not part of the discipline, what is unproved, inconclusive, disordered, or incomprehensible. And everything one says should be well-founded. For all discussions and disputes that are well-founded and clear become a means of healing because they increase the praiseworthy intellect, and an unimpaired intellect leads to the accomplishment of all undertakings.[350]

According to this, discussion does not just enhance a physician's knowledge, making him a better, more efficient doctor, but also benefits him more directly by increasing his intellect, making anything he wishes to undertake easier to achieve.

A number of points here concerning the different goals that can be achieved by discussion deserve further exploration. Caraka defines the first goal from the outset in Ca.Vi.8.6 as the deepening and furthering of a physician's knowledge. This is reiterated in Ca.Vi.8.67, with the additional idea that a physician's intellect is enhanced through debate (as noted). Then, the statement that "discussion with specialists promotes perseverance in and competition for knowledge" implies a goal that goes beyond the more personal interests of the physician: the pursuit of truth. Here, true knowledge is an ideal in itself. The respect for real knowledge and the wish to promote it are evident from the description of friendly debate, in which physicians discuss topics with sincerity and clarity, asking questions and not holding back information. Hostile debate, on the other hand, is only to take place with inferior debate partners, that is, persons whose knowledge is incomplete and deficient. It therefore serves to eradicate false knowledge.

Theoretically, these discussions took place between graduated physicians, but it is possible that students sat in on the debates or even participated—Caraka, after all, notes that one of the benefits of the debates is that a teacher who would only gradually give information to a student might give away secrets in a heated discussion. This benefit seems to be directed at students rather than at graduated physicians, unless we think of it in terms of specialist knowledge that is specific to a particular school (or the teacher's personal secret knowledge) and not to others. What I find particularly important here, however, is the implication of doubt, of incompleteness or even incorrectness of knowledge of some physicians. Although this is perhaps meant to be remedied through the exercise of discussion, the general implication is that some physicians, though they are graduates who are already practicing, may not be fully up to the task. At the same time, these physicians are not necessarily quacks. After all, they are taking part in a formal setup of collegial exchange, which they would have avoided if they were frauds, according to Caraka's definition of quacks in Ca.Sū.29.9.[351] These physicians, then, do not quite fit the profile of the paradigmatic physician who, as one of the four pillars of treatment, "has accurately studied the precepts and principles of the subject, has observed its practice and practiced himself."[352] A medical student's training is meant to be thorough, and a graduate should be able to hold his own in a discussion. However, the fact that a graduate's knowledge may be incomplete is not necessarily due to a deficiency in his education but is linked with the vast amounts of knowledge that can be attained. After all, Caraka states in Ca.Vi.8.14 that "the limits of Ayurveda are indeed not easily passed" and that a diligent person should therefore always keep in constant practice. Although his knowledge is unlikely to be complete, the continuing pursuit of it ensures that a physician rightly belongs in the ranks of respected professionals. But what about the implications of incomplete knowledge for medical practice?

Caraka describes in Vi.8.86 how failure can be avoided through proper training, as well as through self-examination, and through questioning one's abilities before embarking on the treatment of others:

> A physician, then, is one who heals, who is conversant with the meaning and the practical application of the aphoristic rules and by whom life is understood entirely and exactly. And he, desiring to establish the normal state of the humors, should at first examine himself alone, observing the performance of treatments according to the property of the objects, and [asking himself] "Am I capable of carrying out this work or not?"

The question remains what course of action he would take if he came to the conclusion that he was not, in fact, capable of carrying out the work. However, asking the question alone implies that he would not carry out a procedure if he found himself incapable of it. The wider implications of this—that is, whether this would necessitate a return to studies, or perhaps just a meeting with peers, are left unanswered by Caraka.

4

To Care or Not to Care

IN THE BEGINNING of the *Carakasaṃhitā*, the origins of medicine are described in mythological terms.[353] These origins are set in an ancient past, at a time of transition. A perfect, disease-free world, in which all beings lead a long, virtuous life, has transformed into a lesser, tainted world, in which the pursuit of virtuous living—and indeed life itself—has become impeded by illness. There is no explanation why disease suddenly arises, and no moral justification. Disease simply seems to come into being just as everything else in the material world has come into existence. Its arising is therefore value-free. Its moral implications for human life, however, are serious.

A group of sages assemble to discuss the impact of disease on human beings and how to deal with it. Apparently unaffected by disease themselves, the sages feel compassion for the plight of the other sentient beings. Their compassion is not only directed at the bodily discomforts caused by illness, but at the wider implications of disease as an impediment to virtuous living. The sages give some thought to this problem and decide to seek help from Indra (the preeminent god of the Vedic pantheon), from whom they receive an exposition of Ayurveda. Summarizing what they have learnt, the sages then compose the medical treatises for the benefit of mankind.

The spirit in which medical knowledge is transmitted is one of kindness, and the motivation to seek it in the first place one of compassion, the wish to alleviate suffering and to create ideal conditions for virtuous living.[354] As the first human physicians, the sages of this mythic history function as role models. Their attitude of kindness and compassion is exemplary in every sense. And yet, the idea of compassion and kindness—though mentioned several times by some of the medical authors as a virtue in their descriptions of general good conduct (*sadvṛtta*)[355]—is only reiterated once by Caraka as a physician's core characteristic: "Kindness and compassion for those who are ill, affection for the remediable and equanimity toward those in their natural state,[356] this is the quartet of a physician's conduct."[357]

The ethic of kindness and compassion generally comes into question when applied to the subject matter of whom the physician should give medical care to and, more important, whom he should not treat. I have already discussed the kinds of persons a physician is advised not to treat. Two main categories of unwelcome patients emerge from the medical authors' descriptions: (1) social outcasts whom anyone concerned with his reputation would wish to avoid, and (2) persons whose treatment would fail. It is the latter group that is of special interest here, and in particular those patients who suffer from terminal illnesses.

Although physicians are generally advised not to take up treatment of patients diagnosed with terminal illnesses, a closer look into the topic reveals a more differentiated picture. I will discuss the reasons the medical authors give for their advice not to treat terminally ill patients, exploring their guidelines on how a physician may arrive at the decision to avoid or withdraw treatment, and on the exceptions he can make in this process.

To begin with, a physician's decision not to take up or to give up a patient's treatment is meant to be informed. Since he is ideally meant to know all there is to know about disease and cure, his assessment of any medical situation should be accurate, and he would therefore only reject cases for which there exists no cure. His appraisal is based on a complex system of (1) specific signs that warn him of the patient's impending death and (2) disease classification.

The Signs of Impending Death

The ability to recognize the signs that a patient is about to die is part of the good physician's staple requirements: "The entire fruits of Ayurveda are established in one who understands [the subject of] the duration of life. Therefore a physician should indeed always be diligent about knowing the signs of impending death."[358] Significant portions of the medical classics are dedicated to this topic. Caraka, for example, devotes the whole of the Indriyasthāna to the topic of how to recognize the signs that a patient will succumb to his illness, and there are parallel chapters on the signs of impending death in Su.Sū.30–33, Ah.Śā.5–6, As.Śā.9–12, and the Indriyasthāna of the *Kāśyapasaṃhitā*.[359] The signs that foreshadow death are called *riṣṭa* or *ariṣṭa*. They include symptoms displayed by patients, such as particular sudden changes in their physical appearance,[360] or disturbances of the sensory organs: seeing or hearing what is not there, or not seeing or hearing what is there, and changes in the perception of smells and tastes, as well as of touch.[361] Then there are other signs that go beyond the patient's physical symptoms: Strange behavior, particular dreams coupled with physical symptoms, even aberrations in a person's shadow may all point to a patient's approaching death.[362] Finally, some fatal signs are not even displayed by the patients themselves. A physician may, for example, indirectly learn of the patient's imminent death through signs displayed by the persons who come to call him to the patient's home. Everything is significant: the messengers' time of appearance, how they look and behave, as well as the physician's thoughts and actions at the time they arrive, or while he is in contact with them. Further omens may occur on the way to the patient's house, and then again in the patient's house.[363] That these signs are described at such length and in such detail over many chapters shows that it must have been very important indeed for the physician to be able to identify whether a patient would live or not. The descriptions of the signs serve a purpose: they enable the physician to withdraw his services, or to not commence treatment at all, once a patient is diagnosed as incurable. The medical authors are very matter-of-fact about this. Caraka, for example, advises to give up any patient with a terminal illness no fewer than nineteen times in the Indriyasthāna, stating clearly that a physician "should abandon him" (*taṃ parivarjayet*), sometimes even "from afar" (*dūratas, dūrāt*).[364]

Disease Classification

The *ariṣṭa* indicate that a patient will die of his or her illness within a given amount of time, which can span not only hours but also days, weeks, months, and even a year.[365] When a physician decides not to accept a patient or to abandon him on the basis of these signs, the decision is in some sense personal: the *patient* is incurable and must therefore be avoided. However, the classical medical treatises at the same time offer a depersonalized discussion in which not the patient but the *illness* is categorized as curable or as incurable. In line with their conclusion regarding the signs of impending death, the medical authors generally warn not to treat incurable diseases.[366] However, this admonition is not absolute. Caraka explains that there are two types of incurable diseases: those that are unmanageable (*anupakrama*) and those that are controllable (*yāpya*).[367] According to Caraka, diseases categorized as *yāpya* are chronic diseases that do not threaten the patient's life as long as they are managed through diet and regimen.[368] Suśruta makes a distinction between treatable (*kṛtya*) and untreatable (*akṛtya*). He succinctly explains *yāpya* to be an illness of which a patient would die if treatment were withdrawn. The treatment cannot cure the illness but can hold it at bay.[369] Suśruta concludes that one should treat curable diseases, maintain the manageable (though incurable) ones, and reject the incurable ones.[370] This is triage, an important feature of all formal medicine. There are further exceptions to the basic rule of not treating patients afflicted with incurable diseases. Vāgbhaṭa, for example, argues for treatment despite a terminal prognosis as follows:

> Isn't it so that someone who is virtuous and whose life span is fixed will live?[371] Therefore, a physician should treat the patient with care up to his last breath, having informed and obtained the permission of his family and friends.[372]

We will return to this passage when discussing the consequences of treating patients who are fatally ill. However, first we shall turn to the question *why* the medical authors generally advise the physician not to treat the terminally ill.

On the Reasons Not to Treat Terminally Ill Patients

The idea that one's life span is fixed can also be used for the opposite argument: that treatment cannot effect cure because a patient's life span has come to an end (*gatāyus*). Caraka says as much in Ind.11.27: "The four pillars (even when) united and endowed with effective qualities are useless for one whose lifespan has come to an end."

The medical authors give two essential arguments or explanations of why a dying patient should not be treated. The first argument is that treatment would be futile since it would have no effect: the patient's case is hopeless. The medical authors explain the ineffectiveness of medical treatment not merely as a result of the end of an allotted life span, but as an effect of active intervention by hostile entities. Vāgbhaṭa, for example, warns that "one who is dying is approached by Yama's messengers and demons and so on, which destroy the potency of medicines. Therefore one should abandon him."[373]

Note that this argument does not even allow for the possibility of palliative care for the dying, that is, any form of treatment that concentrates on reducing the severity of disease symptoms rather than striving to halt, delay, or reverse progression of the disease itself or provide a cure. It seems that the line of reasoning is that since nothing can be done, nothing should be done.

The second argument or explanation pertains to the consequences failed treatment would have for the physician. As in their statements regarding treating those who are in some sense socially unacceptable, the medical authors maintain that treating a terminally ill patient would damage a physician's reputation. Caraka, for example, explains that "were a physician to treat an incurable disease, he would inevitably suffer the loss of wealth, knowledge, and renown and would meet with censure and rejection."[374] Cakrapāṇidatta refers to this passage in his comment on Caraka's last statement in his four-pillar definition (Ca.Sū.9.26) regarding a physician's detachment from those who are approaching death. Cakrapāṇidatta says: "In this case, indifference is necessary; under this circumstance, medicine should not be administered, and so on, for fear of damaging one's reputation."[375] In another place, Caraka notes that a physician who attends upon a patient "whose strength, flesh, and blood are too depleted, who is afflicted with an incurable disease, and who shows the signs of impending death ... gets saddled with a bad reputation."[376] Suśruta gives equal warning: "By treating someone whose life span has come to an end one would suffer failure in society. Hence, a skilled physician should observe the signs of impending death with care."[377] There is one dissenting voice on this topic: Discussing As.Śā.7.29–31, which recommends that a terminally ill patient should be treated up to his last breath, the commentator Indu states that a physician need not worry about damaging his reputation.[378] This, however, is the exception to the general rule.

Strong social forces seem to be at work here: a bad reputation, censure and rejection, failure in society, and loss of wealth, knowledge, and renown. Note that the reasons given for not treating terminally ill patients are all about the consequences for the physician, while no reasons are given that refer to the patient's welfare. There are a number of possible explanations why treating someone about to die could be seen as a disreputable action. For example, if treatment could not but fail, it could be seen as an unnecessary harassment of the helpless patient. It could also be argued that treatment would incur pointless costs, and that false hopes of recovery would be raised in the patient and those close to him. However, none of these reasons are explored by the medical authors or their commentators. Instead they frame this topic as a discourse on career advice, as it were. From the physician's point of view, treating the moribund must fail, and this means the physician was unsuccessful. Success and failure are absolute terms, with success equalling cure, and thus fame and wealth for the physician, and failure equalling the patient's lingering illness at best, and death at worst, either of which entails a bad reputation and perhaps loss of livelihood for the physician.

A License to Care

While lingering illness despite treatment would have reflected badly on the physicians's abilities, the death of the patient, if interpreted as the direct consequence of the physician's treatment, could lead to punishment. We know from Kauṭilya's *Arthaśāstra* that different punishments were meted out to physicians whose patients died or were injured during treatment.[379] Physical deformity or damage to vital organs was punished in the same way as for causing similar physical injuries through assault.[380] The death of a patient incurred the lowest standard fine, whereas death due to wrong treatment incurred the middle standard fine. Interestingly, these punishments only pertained to physicians who had not reported to the king that they were going to give dangerous treatments, so the offense seems to have been not so much the damage done to the patient as the nondisclosure to the authorities.

Suśruta notes that a physician entering the profession should be licensed, or authorized (*rājānujñāta*) by the king.[381] He also writes that dangerous surgical procedures must be authorized by the king before one undertakes them.[382] Caraka describes the necessity of asking permission of both the authorities and the patient's relatives and friends when a physician is about to embark on a risky procedure:

> In the case of an abdominal disorder [involving] the three humors that is resistent to treatment and does not subside, the physician, voicing doubt, should take action after having asked permission from close relatives, together with friends, the wife, brahmins, kings, and preceptors [*guru*]. He should say: "If no action is taken death is certain, if action is taken there is danger," and if he is authorized by his friends, he should administer him poison mixed with food and drink, or in a fruit in which an angered snake should release its venom.[383]

This scenario describes a last refuge solution to an extreme situation, and is probably not part of standard procedure for medical practice. The therapeutic use of snake poison is certainly unusual: Snake poison is usually dealt with as something a patient needs to be treated for.[384] However, we find a similar prescription in the *Suśrutasaṃhitā* (Cik.14.8), which states that a patient who has taken the poison either dies or recovers from the abdominal disease.

Pointing out the risks of such a drastic treatment and then asking for the authorities' and the relatives' permission to proceed with it is a fail-safe to contain damage to the physician's career if his medical treatment fails and the patient dies. However, it is notable that despite foreseeable problems for the physician, Caraka would still have him undertake this dangerous treatment. This in itself speaks of a certain confidence in the efficacy of the therapy. It is also a testament to Caraka's moral expectation of a physician, namely that a physician must try his absolute best to heal his patient, even if this means embarking on a dangerous course of action with potential difficulties arising for him consequently.

In conclusion, the physician's basic dictum is to not accept patients he cannot cure. This is a rule with a number of exceptions: He can accept patients whose illnesses, though incurable, can be managed. He can also make the decision to continue treating the patient despite knowing that he cannot effect cure with his treatments. This decision may be subject to the permission of the patient's relatives or of other authorities (though seemingly not of the patient himself). What might be perceived as a rather harsh and unforgiving rule is counterbalanced by the underlying assumption that the physician will do his absolute best for the patient. The physician's decision not to treat a patient should be based on his informed and accurate assessment of the case. And since the medical authors greatly emphasize that a physician's medical education and skills should be comprehensive, a physician's ability to treat should encompass all that it is possible to do within the framework of medicine. His giving up a patient, then, may be done in a spirit of self-interest, but it is at the same time based on his realistic knowledge of the limits of medicine.

5

The Rewards of Medical Practice

> Is the physician, taken in that strict sense of which you are speaking, a healer of the sick or a maker of money? And remember that I am now speaking of the true physician.
>
> —Plato, *The Republic*

I HAVE BRIEFLY touched on the topic of the pecuniary relationship between patient and physician.[385] To recapitulate: Wealth is mentioned as one of the characteristics of the ideal patient by several of the medical authors. It is therefore tempting to assume that this particular requirement of the patient is linked to the physician's wish for an income. This suspicion deepens on finding that a healthy person is marked by his having "considerable amounts of money," coupled with "devotion to physicians."[386] Yet further research into this topic shows that the medical authors do not discuss a patient's wealth or lack of it in terms of his ability to remunerate the physician, but rather in terms of his ability to afford the necessary equipment (*upakaraṇa*) or provisions, including medicines for therapy.[387] That a poor person could not afford to pay the physician for his services is not mentioned at all. Instead, the commentators reason that there would be no point in taking up treatment that could not be followed through. This explanation moves responsibility away from the physician and onto the patient. The possibility of charitable treatment—that the physician could not just treat the patient but also supply him with the necessary medicines, and so on—is not discussed in these instances. However, Caraka notes in Sū.15.19–21 that treatments can be modified to suit a smaller purse:

> However, a poor person who has fallen into misfortune may take an appropriate purificatory drug even without having arranged for the desired equipments that are difficult to obtain. For not all men have all the requisite means, nor do severe illnesses not befall the poor. Therefore, in the case of misfortune, whatever medicine can be made by a person should be used as far as possible, as well as clothes and foods.

Caraka also states in Sū.29.9 that it is typical of frauds posing as doctors to "point out that it was the patient himself who lacked equipment, helpers, and the right attitude," when their treatments failed.[388] This places the onus squarely on the physician.

Vāgbhaṭa states in As.Utt.50.192 that the physician should use his own resources to treat the poor.[389] It should also be remembered that Suśruta gives a list of persons whom a physician should treat "with one's own medicine like one's relatives" in Sū.2.8, and this includes a number of persons who clearly would not be able to afford medicines on their own.[390] Both these passages suggest that Suśruta and Vāgbhaṭa expected a physician to be wealthy enough to be able to afford such acts of charity as a matter of course. In any case, the medical authors agree that a physician should be equipped with the instruments and medicines he needs for treatments.[391] While there is no mention of quantities, we can assume that sufficient amounts as needed for treatments are meant. All of this begs the question where the funds to furnish a physician with the necessary equipment and to allow him to treat some patients for free come from. Caraka provides a partial answer in Sū.30.29:[392]

> And it [Āyurveda] should be studied by brahmins, by those of the governing classes [*kṣatriya*], and those of the trade classes [*vaiśya*]: As a favor by brahmins, in order to protect by those of the governing classes, and for a livelihood by those of the trade classes, and generally by all of them to attain virtue, wealth, and pleasure. It is one's highest virtue [*dharma*] to become one who strives to cure the illnesses of those who know metaphysics, of those who practice virtue or of those who expound on virtue, of one's parents, brothers and sisters, relatives, and preceptors, and to contemplate the metaphysical precepts of Ayurveda, to teach them, and to conform to them. Again, it is one's wealth [*artha*] to get money and protection on account of providing health among lords or wealthy persons, and to protect from illness the beings under one's care. Further, it is one's pleasure [*kāma*] to enjoy renown through the acknowledgment of the wise,[393] [their] protection, respect, and service, and to give health to those dear to one.[394]

From this it would seem that, first, it was physicians from a *vaiśya* background who would practice medicine as a trade, while those from brahmin or *kṣatriya* backgrounds would practice for free. Second, whoever the physician, services were meant to be provided for free to relatives, preceptors, and spiritual teachers and those engaged in the study of metaphysics. This squares up nicely with Suśruta's list of persons to treat for free in Sū.2.8 (i.e., the twice-born, teachers, the poor, friends, mendicants, one's dependents, respectable persons, orphans). Finally, the paying clients are identified: lords and wealthy persons. Their patronage could take the form of money, but also of protection. However, it is not clear whether Caraka envisaged a direct transaction between patient and physician, that is, that the physician received payment directly from the patient for each treatment, or a patronage system in which the physician would get financial or other support from patrons that was not subject to specific treatments having taken place and may have allowed him to give treatments to persons other than his patrons.

While physicians from a *vaiśya* background may have earned a livelihood from medicine, there is also some evidence that the *vaiśya* community contributed to medical care through charity:

> In the fifth century C.E., the Chinese Buddhist pilgrim Fa-hsien related that at the city of Pāṭaliputra heads of Vaiśya families established houses for dispensing charity and medicine, to which the poor, the destitute, the maimed, the crippled, and the diseased could resort and receive every kind of help and where physicians would examine their diseases. They obtained the food, medicines, and decoctions they required and were made to feel at ease. When they recovered, they departed.[395]

This does not tell us whether the physicians who examined diseases were on a payroll or gave treatment for free. However, it seems likely that they received payment for their services in this setup.

We know from Kauṭilya's *Arthaśāstra* (2.1.7) that physicians could receive land from the country's ruler to support them:

> He should grant [lands] to priests, preceptors, chaplains, and Brahmins learned in the Vedas [as] gifts to brahmins, exempt from fines and taxes, with inheritance passing on to corresponding heirs, [and] to heads of departments, accountants, and others, and to *gopas*, *sthānikas*, elephant-trainers, physicians, horse-trainers, and couriers, [lands] without the right of sale or mortgage.[396]

K.A.5.3.12 also mentions the figure two thousand as payment for physicians (along with chariot-fighters, elephant-trainers, horse-tamers, carpenters, and animal-breeders) accompanying the army on a military expedition.[397] It is not clear, however, what commodity this number signifies.

There is also some epigraphical evidence of land grants and other payments for physicians: The inscription on the Viṣṇu temple of Veṅkateśa-Perumāḷ at Tirumukkūḍal[398] gives detailed lists of salaries for the staff of a hospital, recording rewards in rice, in money, and in land for the head physician, as well as rewards in rice and in money for medical personnel, including a surgeon.

> 1 tūṇi, 5 *uri* of paddy for 1 kuṟuṇi and 7 nāḻi of rice for feeding 15 in-patients at the rate of 1 nāḻi each, 3 kuṟuṇi of paddy and 8 kāśu per day to Savarṇan Kodaṇḍarāman Aśvatthāma-Bhaṭṭan of Ālappākkam who had obtained land to be enjoyed by himself and his descendants, for prescribing medicines to the patients lying in the hospital. . . . 1 kuṟuṇi of paddy per day to one who performed surgical operations, 2 kuṟuṇi and 2 kāśu per day to 2 persons, at 1 kuṟuṇi and 1 kāśu each, that gathered medicinal herbs, supplied fuel and attended to the preparation of medicines, 1 kuṟuṇi and 1 kāśu per day to 2 nurses, at 4 nāḻi of paddy and 1/2 kāśu each, that attended on the patients and administered medicines.[399]

According to this inscription, patients were provided with food from the funds donated by the hospital's sponsor, King Rājakeśarivarman. Since the inscription names salaries for persons who provided and processed medicines, we can also assume that patients received medicines for free during their stay as well. Note that the dealing with medicines is listed as service rather than as a trade: the persons gathering and processing medicines did not sell the medicines to the hospital but were employed as hospital staff to collect them, and so on.

The list of rewards gives a sense of hierarchy, with the physician Savarṇan Kodaṇḍarāman at the top of the pecking order and the nurses at the bottom. It is interesting to note the distinction between the physician's work (prescribing medicines) and that of the surgeon (performing surgical operations): The physician's work requires theoretical knowledge; the surgeon's work calls for manual skills. The fact that the surgeon received lower pay not only than the physician but also than the persons responsible for medicines and fuel suggests that there was quite a big difference in rank between the surgeon and the physician. This clear division in labor and skills is at odds with the tradition that Suśruta describes, where the ideal physician is one who unites theoretical knowledge with manual skill and the surgeon enjoys the status of respected physician.

The physician depicted in Fa-hsien's travel report and in the inscription seems to have been an employee within a hospital setup. According to the inscription, he had a regular income as well as the benefits of his land grant. On the other hand, the physician in the *Arthaśāstra* seems to have worked independently, and in that respect resembled the physician we know from the medical classics more closely.[400] He may have received a land grant to live from, but we do not learn about other sources of income. Note then that none of these sources connect a physician's livelihood with fees collected from patients. If a physician received money for his services, it was sourced elsewhere.

As already noted, Caraka suggests that the patient always owes a debt to the physician.[401] We find a similar note in the *Bhāvaprakāśa*, which suggests not only that a patient owes a physician for his treatment, but that some sort of transfer from him to the physician would be inevitable: "One who does not recompense for bodily treatment is a fool: The physician gets [the benefit of] each good deed he does."[402] Although Caraka recognizes the obligation of the patient to the physician, he at the same time offers an unequivocal moral evaluation of practicing medicine as a trade, when he states that "those who practice for the sake of a livelihood, selling medical treatment as a trade, are devoted to a heap of dust, having abandoned gold."[403] And yet this does not necessarily mean that a physician should not receive money for his work, but rather that receiving money should not be his primary motivation for undertaking treatment. Bhāvamiśra, for example, admonishes that medicine should not be practised as a trade out of greed but accepts that a physician may receive payment from the wealthy to earn a livelihood.[404] He also lists money (*dravya*) as one of seven essential components of medicine.[405] Wealth is generally understood to be a positive value by the medical authors, and earning a livelihood is recommended to everyone as part of good conduct (*sadvṛtta*).[406] In Ca.Sū.11.5, wealth is described as one of three desires that humans should pursue, the other two being the desire for life and the desire for the other world. Here, Caraka defines earning a livelihood as a duty:

> Then, second, one should pursue the desire for wealth. Next to life, it is wealth that must be striven after. Hence, there is nothing worse than the sin of having a long life without a means of subsistence. For this reason, one should make efforts to strive after means of livelihood.[407]

Generally, wealth appears in the medical classics as one of three, or four, goals of life, the *puruṣārtha*: *artha*, *kāma*, *dharma*, and *mokṣa*: wealth, pleasure, virtue, and spiritual emancipation. Several chapters in the medical treatises end with stating that a physician who practices medicine correctly will attain these goals of life.[408] However, the goal of virtue takes precedence over the goal of wealth, as well as that of pleasure. Caraka makes this abundantly clear:

> A diligent physician, on the other hand, who desires unsurpassed virtue, should save all patients from pain as if they were his own sons. Ayurveda

was revealed by the great sages who, intent on virtue, desired an imperishable state for the sake of religious merit, wealth, and pleasure.[409] One who practises medicine out of compassion toward all creatures rather than for wealth or pleasure overcomes all.[410]

"For someone being dragged into death's realm by savage diseases, no benefactor, either religious or worldly, can match the person who holds out life. There is no gift to compare with the gift of life. The practitioner of medicine who believes that his highest calling is the care of others achieves the highest happiness. He fulfills himself."[411]

Here, Caraka equates compassion with virtue, indeed replaces virtue with compassion as one of three goals of life. He proclaims the care of others to be the physician's highest happiness and fulfilment. This links this passage with Caraka's definition of the four-pillars, where he states that "kindness and compassion for those who are ill" are essential characteristics of the good physician.[412] Within the four-pillar definition, this statement was the exception to the prevailing emphasis on the physician's skill and knowledge as his first and foremost prerequisites. Here, compassion is at the center of Caraka's ethic.

Finally, we may refer to the *Bhāvaprakāśa*, in which the different rewards of medicine are summarized as follows: "Moreover, the reward of medicine is in some cases considered to be wealth, in others friendship, or virtue, or fame, or the practice of medical treatment; thus medicine is never without reward."[413]

To conclude, the classical medical treatises are, broadly speaking, silent on the question how a physician made his living. We can glean a little information from Caraka, who suggests that physicians from a *vaiśya* background may practice for money and protection from lords and wealthy persons. Evidence from other sources points to a patronage system in which physicians were awarded land and money for their services, in some cases as employees in a hospital setting.

While the question of fiscal rewards is only partially answered, Caraka offers some insight into another reason a physician might dedicate himself to his work: Because this work offers him the ultimate rewards of happiness, fulfillment, and virtue. Here, medical practice is discussed in terms of a calling rather than a profession, with spiritual and emotional rewards given predominance over material benefits. The physician's ethic of skill and knowledge that is so dominant throughout the medical treatises is in this instance replaced by an ethic of compassion.

Finally, Bhāvamiśra's summary of the rewards of medicine includes wealth, friendship, virtue, and fame and moreover attributes the same value to all of these. He concludes that medical practice never remains without reward.

6

Veracity in the Doctor–Patient Relationship

LAYING OUT Aframework of guidelines for professional ethics, Beauchamp and Childress, the authors of *Principles of Biomedical Ethics*, identify four clusters of moral principles they consider central to biomedical ethics. These are:

1. *Respect for autonomy* (a norm of respecting the decision-making capacities of autonomous persons)
2. *Nonmaleficence* (a norm of avoiding the causation of harm)
3. *Beneficence* (a group of norms for providing benefits and balancing benefits against risks and costs)
4. *Justice* (a group of norms for distributing benefits, risks, and costs fairly)[414]

While the principles of nonmaleficence and beneficence are firmly anchored in historical traditions of Western medical ethics (i.e., the medical ethics that has its roots in the Hippocratic medical traditions and those that developed from them), the principle of respect for autonomy marks a fundamental shift in the history of the doctor–patient relationship from medical paternalism to an emphasis on patient's rights. Medical paternalism, the dominant model of the doctor–patient relationship until well into the second half of the twentieth century, is based on the principle that a doctor should act benignly in accordance with his[415] conception of the patient's needs for treatment, information, and consultation. This model rejects the notion that a patient has a right to information and hence to autonomy in judgment. In practice, this means that it is up to the doctor's discretion whether he will or will not disclose medical information to a patient or a patient's relatives or guardians, and to what extent he will do so. In a paternalistic doctor–patient relationship, the doctor may opt for comprehensive, accurate, and objective information if he judges his patient fit to receive such information. He may, however, also choose the under or nondisclosure of information, or even give false information, depending on the circumstances. Assuming that the doctor–patient relationship is of a fundamentally benign nature, a doctor's well-considered and deliberate choice to give partial or wrong information is perfectly in accord with accepted standards of behavior in the paternalistic model. Speaking untruths, which in other contexts might be seen as morally reprehensible, becomes a correct action of positive moral value.

The Epistemology of Honesty and Lying in the Ayurvedic Classics

In the *Suśrutasaṃhitā*, the relationship between physician and patient is described as one that requires trust on the side of the patient and benevolence on the side of the physician. Suśruta argues as follows:

> A patient may mistrust even his mother, father, children, or relatives but places trust in a doctor. He himself gives himself over, and he does not distrust him. Because of that, the physician ought to protect that patient like a son.[416]

Suśruta here thus postulates a special relationship between doctor and patient in which the patient's trust is justified by the paternal benevolence of the physician. A patient can trust in a physician because a physician is obliged to be benign. Indeed, according to Suśruta's reasoning, it seems that the very act of trust on the patient's side is what obliges the physician to be worthy of that trust.

As we have seen, the medical treatises standardly characterize a good doctor as someone whose professional knowledge and skills are impeccable. A good patient's key characteristic, on the other hand, is his obedience to the doctor. Obedience to the doctor implies trust in the doctor, while the emphasis on the physician's skills serves to establish the physician as one who deserves this trust. Here, then, it is not a physician's attitude toward the patient that makes him worthy of trust but his qualifications as a doctor.

Once the relationship of one who trusts and one who is worthy of trust is established, the balance of power shifts toward the physician. The patient is now meant to voluntarily submit to the physician's judgment, and in some sense to surrender control over his life to the physician. The doctor knows best—at least if he is a good doctor—and he will decide for the patient what needs to be done, while the patient is expected to comply with the doctor's instructions.

In such a top-down relationship between doctor and patient, information management, including under- and nondisclosure, deception, and lying, is a matter of the doctor's discretion. And, as we will see, that is indeed broadly the idea brought forward by the ayurvedic authors, who in some instances advise deception as a legitimate means to shield patients and their relatives from upsetting news; to ensure patient compliance; or even to bring about a certain therapeutic effect. At the same time, however, these authors advocate honesty as a requisite virtue of a good doctor (or a good medical student) in accordance with their general instructions on good conduct (*sadvṛtta*). Caraka, for example, instructs unequivocally *nānṛtaṃ brūyāt*, "One should not lie," in his chapter on good conduct.[417]

General discussions on honesty and dishonesty are usually part of a larger discourse on righteousness and unrighteousness, good and bad conduct, or healthy and unhealthy behaviors, all of which forms the backdrop against which the medical authors delineate the rules for a physician's conduct. Therefore, before we look more closely at the specifics of the role and use of honesty (and of deception or lying) in the doctor–patient relationship, we will examine the wider epistemology of honesty and lying in the ayurvedic texts. The following passages from the *Carakasaṃhitā*, *Suśrutasaṃhitā*, *Aṣṭāṅgahṛdayasaṃhitā*, and *Aṣṭāṅgasaṃgraha* were chosen for their use of such keywords as "truth" (*satya*), falsehood or dishonesty (*anṛta*), and deception (*chadman* and *upadhā*), and their connections with wider contexts.[418]

A passage from the *Carakasaṃhitā* (Ca.Vi.3.24) on the origins of disease may serve as the starting point in our exploration of the meaning of honesty and dishonesty in an ayurvedic epistemology. In this passage, set within the chapter on epidemics,[419] we are projected into a faraway past that stands at the beginning of the transmission of ayurvedic knowledge, as it is passed on from the sage Punarvasu Ātreya to his disciple Agniveśa. In his lesson, Ātreya places the origins of disease in the time of the transition from the Golden Age (*kṛtayuga*) to the next, the Silver Age (*tretāyuga*).[420] During this passage from one age to the next, the condition of humans and their behavior and attitudes undergo changes that transform them from perfect beings and paragons of righteousness to increasingly flawed and unrighteous beings. As one vice spawns the next, righteousness wanes and unrighteousness takes hold of the world:

> At the beginning of the Golden Age, as [the elements], beginning with earth,[421] were full of every good quality, grains with unimaginable properties of savor, potency, postdigestive savor, and specific action arose for those whose nature, qualities, and actions were noble.[422] As the Golden Age came to an end, the bodies of some of those prosperous beings became heavy as they consumed too much. In the Golden Age, weariness developed from this heaviness of body, from weariness laziness, from laziness accumulation, from accumulation possession, and from possession greed. Then, in the Silver Age, malice issued from

> greed, lying from malice, and lust, anger, arrogance, hatred, harshness, violence, fear, sorrow, grief, anxiety, distress, and so on from lying. Then, in the Silver Age, a fourth of righteousness disappeared. Because of its disappearance, there was a decrease by a fourth of the amount of rain in the age. And there was a loss of a fourth of the quality of earth and so on. A decline by a fourth of oiliness, purity, savor, potency, post-digestive savor, and specific action in the grains was caused by this loss. After that, people's bodies, not supported as they used to be through diet and lifestyle, which had lost a fourth of quality, and seized by fire and wind, were from now on overpowered by diseases like fever and so on. From that time, living beings gradually suffered a decrease of life span.

This particular account of the origin of disease is only found in the *Caraka-saṃhitā,* but it introduces a paradigm that is nearly universal to ayurvedic literature: the connection between human action and health and longevity. From the story it appears that human conduct is a decisive element in the prevention or the propagation of disease: While humans act righteously, health and happiness prevail; when they lapse into unrighteous behavior, a chain reaction is started that ends with the spread of disease and reduced life expectancy. Lying forms a prominent part in Caraka's chain of human frailties, as it calls forth a deluge of negative emotions: lust, anger, arrogance, hatred, harshness, violence, fear, sorrow, grief, anxiety, and distress. From there, the downward spiral seems inevitable, particularly since there is no indication of agency on the part of the humans, that is, that they could choose to act or feel one way or another, righteously or unrighteously, truthfully or falsely. Rather, it seems that their vices are simply a symptom of the inherent character of the age and part of a predestined evolutionary development.

The theme of lacking agency or decision-making capacity is echoed in Suśruta's delineations of personality typologies. Using the Sāṃkhya[423] concept of the three *guṇas*, or qualities, Suśruta categorizes persons as *sāttvika* (i.e., endowed with qualities associated with goodness, purity and vigor), *rājasa* (i.e., influenced by the agitating quality of passion), or *tāmasa* (i.e., affected by the qualities of darkness, ignorance, and illusion).[424] Suśruta outlines the human typologies in Śā.1.18 as follows:

> The [qualities] associated with goodness [*sattva*] are benevolence, pleasure in sharing with others, patience, honesty, righteousness, faithfulness, knowledge, intellect, understanding, mindfulness, resolution, and nonattachment. The ones associated with passion [*rajas*] are much unhappiness, a tendency to wandering around, irresoluteness, egotism,

> falsehood, lack of compassion, deceit, arrogance, excitement, lust, and anger. Those associated with darkness [*tamas*] are dejection, nihilism, a tendency to unrighteousness, restraint of the intellect, ignorance, stupidity, a tendency to inactivity, and sleepiness.

This definition delineates an asymmetrical dichotomy with all that is associated with *sattva* on one side and all that is associated with *rajas* or *tamas* on the other. This opposition is expressed by the use of negative prefixes (*dhṛti/adhṛti, jñāna/ajñāna, āstikya/nāstikya*) or of semantically opposed words (*satya/ānṛtikatva*). Several of the characteristics on each side do not have an opposite on the other, like "pleasure in sharing" (*saṃvibhāgarucitā*), associated with *sattva*, or "habit of wandering around" (*aṭanaśīlatā*), associated with *rajas*, or "sleepiness" (*nidrālutva*), associated with *tamas*. However, without having an exact opposite in the other group, these cases still may be understood to express the qualitative difference between the concepts of *sattva* and *rajas/tamas*. It is tempting to order the listed attributes into a framework of good (i.e., belonging to *sattva*) and bad (i.e., belonging to *rajas/tamas*) qualities, as this would allow us to interpret honesty as a good quality by virtue of its association with *sattva*, and dishonesty as a bad quality because of its association with *rajas*. However, Suśruta's categorization is in itself neutral and does not explicitly state moral judgement. And indeed, in a more elaborate list of typologies (Su.Śā.4.75–94) in which Suśruta specifies seven personality types related to *sattva*, six related to *rajas*, and three related to *tamas*, we find attributes in the latter two categories that need not necessarily be judged negative, such as powerful (*aiśvaryavat*) and brave (*śūra*) as markers of the *rajas* personality. Honesty is not featured in this list as a characteristic of a *sattva* disposition. Neither are lying or falsehood listed as part of a *rajas* or *tamas* disposition here. However, another attribute of the same semantic category is found as a defining characteristic of one of the six *rajas* temperaments, the "snake's nature" (*sarpasattva*): being deceitful, or tricky (*māyānvita*).

In the *Carakasaṃhitā* (Śā.4.36–40), we find an analogous list of personality typologies, with seven subcategories of the first type, six that are associated with *rajas* and three associated with *tamas*. The first typology group parallels Suśruta's *sattva* category, but Caraka uses the term *śuddha*, "pure," instead. According to Ca.Sū.1.57–58, *rajas* and *tamas* are the mental parallels (but not correlations) of the bodily *doṣas* wind, bile, and phlegm:

> Wind, bile, and phlegm are called the bodily sum of faults. Both *rajas* and *tamas* again are described as the mental sum of faults. The former one is calmed down by medicines depending on divine and rational

> [measures], the mental one by knowledge, discernment, steadfastness, mindfulness, and meditation.[425]

As H. Scharfe has shown, Caraka generally uses the term *doṣa* in a negative sense, so that by calling *rajas* and *tamas* mental *doṣas*, he defines them as negative qualities.[426] Caraka spells this out even more clearly in Śā.4.34, where he explains that *rajas* and *tamas* spoil the *sattva* (here used in the sense of "the mind").[427]

According to both Caraka and Suśruta, the characteristic tendencies of each personality type become particularly prominent under the influence of intoxicating substances. In line with his general positive/negative categorization of the *guṇas*, Caraka interprets these tendencies as signs of a superior, inferior, or average nature in Cik.24.72–73: "Rain awakens grain and fire shows the nature of gold, but wine does both to all beings. As fire shows the kinds [of gold] to be superior, inferior or average, wine shows the nature of beings to be superior, inferior, or average." This passage is followed by remarks on the typological characteristics of drinking partners, which allows the reader to conclude that Caraka is referring to the respective qualities of each personality type when he classifies persons as superior, inferior, or average.

Suśruta discusses the different reactions typologically different persons display when under the influence of alcoholic or intoxicating beverages (*madya*) in Sū.45.207–209, warning that persons of predominantly *rajas* or *tamas* disposition would be disagreeable drinking partners and should be shunned, if possible. According to Su.Sū.45.209, persons influenced most strongly by the qualities of *tamas* would, among other things, speak untruths when intoxicated: "And in a person affected by the quality of darkness [*tamas*], intoxication would cause uncleanliness, sleep, envy, intercourse with women who should not be approached, wantonness, and lying." Note that in Suśruta's general introduction to the personality types, he lists speaking falsehoods as a characteristic of *rajas* personalities rather than of *tamas* personalities.

Though Caraka and Suśruta have somewhat different interpretations of the meaning and functions of the *guṇas*, they share the fundamental notion that the *guṇas* determine how a person thinks, feels, and acts. Unfortunately, they don't explain how exactly a person comes to have his or her personality type or predominance of one psychological quality—whether they are "genetically" preordained constitutions, determined at conception or birth; or something a person acquires and thus can change during lifetime through lifestyle or mental discipline. Caraka, however, does suggest in Sū.1.57 that mental faults can be remedied through knowledge, discernment, steadfastness, mindfulness, and meditation, and thus advocates agency and choice rather than complete predetermination of human emotion and action. Accordingly, a person of a *rajas* constitution may have an initial tendency or impulse toward lying but can choose not to lie, thereby diminishing the tendency itself.

Human agency and choice are central to ancient Indian medicine, which relies on a person's ability to choose a certain lifestyle, or to act on medical advice (incurable diseases and natural death being the exceptions to this rule, and the only circumstances in which a physician—and any human—must accept defeat). A human's options for actively seeking health and happiness and avoiding the opposite are laid out at length in the context of daily and seasonal regimen (a feature found in most of the ayurvedic classics), as well as in other contexts. The possibility of choice is expressed through the use of the optative in these passages. A person "should" or "ought to" (or "should not" or "mustn't") think, say, or do something, which clearly indicates that any of these activities is a matter of choice. Suśruta (Cik.24.90), for example, gives the following instructions in his chapter on healthy conduct (*svasthavṛtta*):

> One should not speak what is hated by the king, harsh, slanderous, and untrue, nor should one blame gods, brahmins, and ancestors, or serve those who are hated by the king, insane, fallen [from their class], low, and inferior.

The choice implied by the use of the optative verbal mood is not necessarily a moral one, but may be quite utilitarian and meant to bring about more or less tangible results. A number of effects are on offer: happiness, wealth, and pleasure, or—perhaps more appropriate to a medical context—health and longevity. At the beginning of Cikitsāsthāna 44, Suśruta notes specifically that the chapter's instructions are about accomplishing health, indicating that any categorization of what should be done or ought not to be done is first of all based on its implication for health.

A passage in the Carakasaṃhitā (Śā.2.46) confirms the connection between conduct and health:

> A man who resorts to a wholesome diet and lifestyle, who examines [everything] closely, who is not attached to the objects of the senses, who is liberal and impartial, to whom truth is paramount, who is forbearing, and who is devoted to those who are accomplished becomes free from disease. [428]

There are two ways of interpreting this passage. One is that good conduct (i.e., resorting to a wholesome diet, being honest, etc.) leads to or even guarantees health. The other is that the described conduct or lifestyle is not good per se in a moral sense but good in that it is *useful* for attaining or maintaining health. A similar passage in the *Aṣṭāṅgahṛdayasaṃhitā* (Śā.3.120) connects good conduct with the prolongation of life. Here, there is a slight shift in emphasis from utilitarianism to a more moral perspective, as Vāgbhaṭa writes that the outlined conduct is a way to prolong a *virtuous* life, rather than just to prolong life in general: "Charity, good conduct, compassion, truthfulness, celibacy, gratitude, rejuvenative therapies and benevolence form the group that prolong a virtuous life." A different connection between health and conduct is delineated by Caraka in his chapter on the nonsuppression of urges (*na vegān dhāraṇīyam adhyāya*, Ca.Sū.7.26–30), where he defines certain mental or physical actions as urges and explains that how one deals with such impulses has a direct impact on health:

> However, one who desires well-being both in this world and in the next should check those urges of blameworthy recklessness in the actions of mind, speech, and body.[429] A wise person should restrain the urges of greed, grief, fear, anger, and arrogance, of shamelessness, envy, excessive passion, and desire. One should check the urge to speak harshly, excessively, treacherously, falsely, and untimely when it arises. One should restrain urges to [commit] any bodily practice connected with hurting another, like illicit intercourse, theft, violence, and so on. A man who is virtuous in word because he is faultless in the actions of mind, speech, and body is happy and enjoys and accumulates righteousness, wealth, and pleasure.

Again, the aim is well–being, as well as happiness, wealth, and pleasure. Lying is here described as an urge of "blameworthy recklessness," clearly defining it as a negative action that has a definite detrimental effect on health as well as on other aspects of life: It is an urge (and as such innate to every human) that should be suppressed.

To summarize: From the above excerpts, it is clear that the ayurvedic authors understand honesty to be a virtue: a righteous behavior that is useful for maintaining both an individual's and society's health and happiness. A good person is characterized by his adherence to the truth or, more generally, by his honest character. Such a person is likely to have a *sattva* personality, which makes him a superior being altogether. Dishonesty, on the other hand, is associated with the opposite qualities. It leads to a number of negative and hurtful emotions in the first instance, and has negative implications for the health of the individual and that of society. Lying is a characteristic of *tamas* or *rajas* personalities and as such generally an undesirable behavior. In discussions on good conduct, instructions on honesty and dishonesty are unequivocal: one should not lie!

Finally, Caraka's definition of lying as an urge of blameworthy recklessness—probably the strongest statement one can find in the medical classics on this topic—leaves no doubt about whether lying is an unacceptable action. The reasons for its unacceptability may lie in practical consideration rather than in morality, but it is a clear and unambiguous social rule nevertheless.

And yet, as we have indicated in the introduction to this chapter, the medical authors do allow for circumstances in which it would be permissable or even desirable for a physician to lie to his patient. What seemed an absolute rule becomes less absolute and somewhat blurred when applied to the doctor–patient relationship. Here, as we will see in the following section, the concept of honesty pertains to a physician's *character* rather than to his actions, while truth itself is a qualifiable concept.

A Physician's Honesty: Truth, But Not the Whole Truth

There are several contexts in which a physician's honesty is discussed in the medical classics. One of these is the medical student's initiation, descriptions of which are found in the *Suśrutasaṃhitā*, the *Carakasaṃhitā*, the *Aṣṭāṅgahṛdayasaṃhitā*, the *Aṣṭāṅgasaṃgraha* and the *Kāśyapasaṃhitā*, as been discussed in Chapter 2. Suśruta gives particular emphasis to the virtue of honesty in his version of the initiation, calling the student to abandon untruth, and to be totally devoted to truth as part of his studentship.[430]

Caraka mentions honesty twice in his version of the medical student's initiation in Vimānasthāna 8.13. The first instance parallels Suśruta'a passage, relating to a medical student's behavior during his apprenticeship and describing the spartan habits he should adopt while studying with his teacher: "You should lead the austere life of a student, wearing a beard, speaking the truth, not eating meat, resorting to that which is pure, [and] unselfish, and not carrying weapons."[431] The second pertains to the medical student's behavior once he is a practising physician. He then should "speak gently, purely, justly, joyfully, in a wholesome manner, truthfully, affectionately, and moderately."[432]

In the *Kāśyapasaṃhitā* (Vi.2[?].4), truthfulness is listed as one of the desired qualities of a pupil, but it is not mentioned in the same chapter's description of the method of practice. Finally, the *Aṣṭāṅgasaṃgraha*'s summary of the student's initiation (Sū.2.1–7) makes no mention at all of honesty or dishonesty as a virtue required of the student or the practicing physician.

As we have seen, Caraka is alone in demanding honesty of the practicing physician. However, the rule to "speak truthfully" is apparently not absolute, as it is followed by conflicting advice concerning communication with patients in the very same passage: "And even if you know that the life span of the diseased is diminished, you should not tell this in a situation in which by speaking [about it], you would harm the diseased or another."[433] This would seem to imply that Caraka differentiates between lying and withholding the truth. "Speaking truthfully" then means telling the truth, but not necessarily the whole truth. The validity of this concept of truthfulness, however, rests on a crucial assumption: When Caraka advises not to tell all that is to tell, he specifies that the disclosure of information should be subject to the potential damage a patient might suffer from hearing it. This reflects a fundamental paradigm of medical paternalism: beneficence, according to which the consideration of a patient's well-being is central to any communication or interaction between doctor and patient. Under the rules of paternal beneficence, not telling the whole truth in order to shield a patient from harm represents the ethically correct choice of action.

Ensuring Patient Compliance

In the following section, I would like to discuss a more active use of deception or untruth by the doctor as part of his therapeutic method. In the introduction to this chapter, I have stated that the medical authors propose deception as an appropriate course of action to facilitate medical treatment by ensuring patient compliance. A passage from Caraka's Cikitsāsthāna—the section on therapeutics—gives an example of how deception may be used by a physician to make sure that patients get the treatment they need. This passage has already been commented on by Francis Zimmermann in his landmark publication *The Jungle and the Aroma of Meats,* where he discusses it in the context of the tension in the ayurvedic classics between a therapeutic system of purity, based on nonviolence, abstinence, and vegetarianism, and a therapeutic system of force and virility, in which a certain amount of violence exists through the use of meat, purging, and so on. Counter to what one might expect from texts that position themselves within a brahmanic context, now widely associated with vegetarianism,[434] the early classical medical treatises present the use of meat, either as part of diet, or as part of a medicinal preparation quite casually and do not discuss it at all as an ethical issue vis-à-vis vegetarianism or other food rules.[435]

Ca.Cik.8. is about therapies against consumption or wasting disease, and the passage that is relevant to our discussion provides the reader with a list of meats that are declared particularly nourishing and strengthening for those who are emaciated and worn out. The catch is that what is considered the most nourishing type of meat by Caraka—the meat of meat-eaters (*māṃsādamāṃsa*)—seems to have also been regarded as an unacceptable food by his contemporaries. Thus, Caraka warns the reader that patients may refuse to eat this meat or may vomit when told what it was. To avoid this, he advises the physician to deceive the patient by presenting the carnivore's meat as the meat of a more acceptable animal and provides a list of replacement names:

> One who knows the rules should give those who are dehydrated and whose flesh is wasting the prepared meat of meat-eaters, which is particularly nourishing. To one who is dehydrated, he should give peacock and other [meats] under the name of peacock: vulture, owl, and blue jay, well-prepared according to the rules. He should give crows under the name of partridge, and fried snakes under the name of fish; as well as earthworms under the name of fish entrails. A physician should give cooked jackals, large mongooses, cats, and young jackals under the name of hare. To increase flesh, he should give lions, bears and hyenas, tigers, and meat-eaters of such a kind under the name of antelope. To increase flesh, the doctor should give the seasoned[436] meat of elephant, rhinoceros, and horse in the name of buffalo. Valued for [its] pungent, hot, and light [properties], the meat of particular kinds of beasts and birds whose bodies are abundantly covered in meat is the best provider of flesh.

Caraka concludes:

> He should employ deception about those meats that aren't liked because [they are] unusual, because that way they can be eaten easily. Knowing [what it was], feeling disgusted, [the patient] would not even eat, or would cause what was eaten to come up again. Therefore, he should let such meats be administered after they have been disguised.

This practical advice is echoed by Vāgbhaṭa in Ah.Cik.5.7:

> [The meat of] vultures and birds of prey, donkeys, and camels is wholesome when prepared so as to be unrecognizable; when recognized, it is abhorred and therefore [would cause] vomiting instead of strength and vigor.

Note how neither Caraka nor Vāgbhaṭa mentions beef, which is now the kind of meat an orthodox Hindu and particularly a brahmin would absolutely avoid.[437]

Suśruta also devotes a similar passage to the treatment of consumption, which he calls *śoṣa* rather than *rājayakṣma*. Su.Utt.41.35–36 and 39 have direct reference to the preparation of carnivores, as well as of some other animals. While Suśruta here does not, like Caraka, advise the physician to give particular meats under other names, he does hint at using deception when giving certain meats in Utt.41.35: "One should give [the meat of] crows, owls, mongooses, cats, earthworms, beasts of prey, hole-dwellers and moles, and vultures *under various pretexts*, fried in mustard oil with rock salt." Suśruta has more to say about the meat of meat-eaters in Cik.1.82cd–83ab, where he discusses it in the context of treating patients with wounds. Here, the meat of meat-eaters is said to promote the growth of flesh—probably for covering deep wounds: "A man should eat meats of meat-eaters according to rule. The flesh of one whose mind is pure grows through meat." Ḍalhaṇa, Suśruta's commentator, specifies meat-eaters such as lions and so on. He also explains "one whose mind is pure" (*viśuddhamanas*) as "one whose mind is not beset by sorrow, anger, and so on" but adds that the commentator Jejjaṭa interprets *viśuddhamanas* differently: "The meats of lions and so on are given under disguise, thus 'of one whose mind is pure.' "[438] Jejjaṭa's comment, as quoted by Ḍalhaṇa, links Suśruta's passage on the treatment of wounds and Caraka's passage on the treatment of *rājayakṣma* by bringing terms into context that are not actually common to these passages (i.e., *viśuddhamanas* occurs only in the *Suśrutasaṃhitā*, and *chadmopahita* only in the *Carakasaṃhitā*).[439]

When Caraka writes that one should give patients meats under false names, he explains that persons will not want to eat something that they are not used to (*anabhyāsa*). Caraka's commentator Cakrapāṇidatta brings this matter to a more complex level, when he glosses *anabhyāsa*, "lack of habit," with *abhakṣyatva*, "not to be eaten," a technical term found in reference to food laws of brahmanic law literature.[440] And indeed, most of Caraka's items fall into the categories of forbidden foods found in Manu's Dharmaśāstra. Manu's categories also include animals that are not meat-eaters. This could explain why Caraka mentions horses and elephants in a list otherwise consisting of carnivores.[441] Caraka's list of meats also corresponds to a list found in the rules of discipline for Buddhist monks in the Pāli Canon (Vinayapiṭaka, Suttavibhaṅga, Pacittiya 8.4). If the meats listed by Caraka were subject to food laws his contemporaries generally adhered to, their use in therapy would have serious ethical implications. Patients might, for example, consider themselves irredeemably spiritually tainted by the use of such substances—or they might understand it as a minor misdemeanor, easily expiated. Intentionality might play a role in establishing whether an offense was committed: It might make a difference that the patients did not know what they were taking.[442] Finally, the physician might be considered tainted by administering impure food, either through being in contact with it or by committing a bad deed through making someone else take such a food. This discussion goes beyond either Caraka's or Cakrapāṇidatta's treatment of the subject.[443] This omission is somewhat surprising, given that diet is such a central concern in Ayurveda. An acknowledgment and debate of existing food laws would therefore prima facie seem a necessity. Yet Caraka's prescriptive menu of meats not only runs completely counter to brahmanic prohibitions but does this quite casually. What made such a cavalier attitude possible? It is conceivable that the religious food rules mentioned were simply of no particular importance to the society Caraka (or later Cakrapāṇidatta) lived and worked in.

A comment made by Cakrapāṇidatta in a different context (*at* Ca.Sū.8.29) may give a clue to why religious prohibitions may have been disregarded by Caraka: "For the rules of ayurveda do not teach the achievement of righteousness. Rather, they teach the achievement of health."[444] However, the medical authors, and Caraka among them, do on many occasions display both a knowledge of and, more important, agreement with brahmanic customs,[445] and the correspondence of Caraka's list of foods to foods forbidden by Manu (or by the Buddhist Canon) is too extensive to be coincidental. Perhaps the question is which came first: the custom not to eat certain foods (and remember, it is that the meats are "uncustomary," *anabhyāsa*, that Caraka refers to) or the brahmanic (or Buddhist) prohibition? Unfortunately, this question cannot be answered here, so we are left only with the observation that it does not seem Caraka's intention to link his choice of prescribed meats with religious significance or deeper meaning.

To return to the initial topic of deception, it should be noted that the passage in Caraka's Cikitsāsthāna 8 is not composed as an ethical discourse in general. While it indicates that a physician may need to make allowances for a patient's attitude or feelings toward a substance—a concern that is rarely expressed in the medical texts—it does not present this as an ethical dilemma for the physician, but simply as a matter for practical consideration. Caraka is not asking moral questions about truthfulness or whether a physician should give a substance to patients that they object to. He simply promotes deception as a tool to ensure patient compliance. However, Caraka's commentator Cakrapāṇidatta questions the moral implications of Caraka's practical advice and compares it with a statement Caraka makes in a passage on good conduct (*sadvṛtta*) in another part of his work (Ca.Sū.8.19). There, Caraka states "one should not tell a lie" (*nānṛtaṃ brūyāt*), which leads Cakrapāṇidatta to ask whether this does not contradict what is said in Cikitsāsthāna 8.19: that one should use deception (*upadhā*) in saying that one animal's meat is that of another. He answers his own question as follows:

> "One should not lie" should not be seen as a contradiction to the advice about speaking falsely beginning with "crows by the name of partridge" and so on in the context of royal consumption, since the guilt of speaking falsehood is incurred by speaking untruth that results in harming another, but not by speaking untruly for the sake of another's life.[446]

In other words, truth, or rather untruth, can be morally qualified. It is only a vice when used to harm others, and is acceptable when used for a good cause. Thus, tricking a patient into using a substance that is medically efficacious, albeit generally considered disgusting, is an act not of vice but of virtue. The underlying principle here is that whatever needs to be done to ensure patient compliance—always a key factor for the success of any therapy—may, or indeed should, be done.

We have seen how ayurvedic authors advise deception as a legitimate means to shield patients and their relatives from upsetting news, as well as to ensure patient compliance. I will now explore a third possibility: the use of deception as a tool to bring about a certain therapeutic effect.

Deception as a Therapeutic Tool

In Cikitsāsthāna 9, Caraka describes various types of madness (*unmāda*) and their treatment. For patients who suffer from madness categorized as *paittika*—associated with the humor, *pitta*, or bile—Caraka prescribes the following ways of interacting with the patient as part of the therapy:

> Or a friend should encourage him with words of religious merit and wealth, or tell him of the death of a beloved one, or show him startling things. Or, after he has been fettered and oiled with mustard oil, one should lay him down stretched out on the back in the sun. Or one should touch him with velvet bean [*kapikacchu*],[447] or with heated metal, oil, or water. Or, having struck him with whips, one should confine him firmly fettered in a deserted house, for his confused mind thus comes to rest. One should scare him with a snake whose fangs have been extracted, or with tamed lions[448] and elephants, or with robbers or enemies holding knives. Or otherwise, royal officers should take the well-restrained [patient] outside and should scare him, threatening to

> kill him on the king's order.[449] For the fear for one's life is thought to exceed fears of bodily pain. Through this his disordered mind comes to rest.[450]

Ah.Utt.6.48–51, As.Utt.9.54–57, and Bhāv.Madh.8.22.39–42 copy Caraka's instructions, quoting him nearly verbatim, the former two with one variant reading each at the same place: Caraka's *trāsayeyur* ("they should scare") in Cik.9.83 is replaced with *bhāpayeyur*, "they should intimidate," in the *Aṣṭāṅgahṛdayasaṃhitā*, and again with another word in the *Aṣṭāṅgasaṃgraha*: *bheṣayeyur*, "they should make fear." This scenario points to such treatments taking place in a courtly setting, or at least in proximity to it. This is indicated not only by the role royal officers (or persons disguising as such) play in it but also by the use of such animals as lions and elephants. These, and the lion in particular, would hardly have been easily available to normal citizens.[451]

However, the treatments themselves stand in striking contrast to privileges one might associate with a courtly setting, as—apart from the initial suggestion that "a friend should encourage him with words of religious merit and wealth"—they are characterized by various degrees of violence to the patient. A low level of violence lies in the telling of sad news. These may be quite untrue, but—true or not—are probably intended to let the patient experience anguish or strong grief. Whipping, burning, fettering, and isolating the patient are more marked displays of violence. However, the central method of treatment is the use of threat. Each threat—of being bitten by a snake, attacked by lions or elephants, assaulted by robbers or enemies, or executed by royal officers on the king's orders—is aimed at making the patient fear for his life. However, Caraka indicates fairly clearly that these threats are just that: the patient is at no time in real danger of losing his life. After all, the snake's fangs should have been removed and the lions and elephants should be tame. As for the robbers and enemies, it is very unlikely that true criminals were at the physician's disposal, so that we can safely assume that some chosen persons were to play-act, pretending to be robbers with the intention of assaulting the patient with knives. The same goes for the execution threats of the royal officers, whether real or not. As there is no true intention of seriously harming the patient, the threat is in fact an act of deception. The treatment's success relies on the contrasting perspectives the participants in this medical drama have: While the doctor/carer/royal officer does not intend to actually commit the violent act or to let it happen, it is crucial that the patient believes he does. The violent fear that the patient experiences is what is meant to ultimately set his mind (which, as we must remember, is disturbed, as he is mentally ill) to rest. However, the actual mental processes that bring on this change are unfortunately not explained by Caraka, who merely points out that the fear for one's life is an extremely powerful emotion, stronger even than the fear of bodily pain.

Similar treatments are described by Suśruta in Utt.62.17–21b:

> One should show him startling things, or tell him about the death of one dear to him. One should intimidate him with men of fearful appearance, with tamed elephants and poisonless snakes. Or one should then beat him with whips, after he has been fettered with chains. Or, having restrained him, one should frighten the well-guarded one with a grass-fire. Or else one should threaten him with water, or one should pretend [to threaten him] with blows with a rope. And a strong man should guard him, and make him stand overnight in water. One should pierce him with a pointed tool [*āra/ā*, awl], [but] one should avoid injuring the vital points [*marman*]. Having entered a house, one should set that house on fire, protecting him. Or one should constantly keep him in a covered and waterless pit well.

Suśruta's suggestions for treatment are an even more startling read than Caraka's, though the basic principle is the same: deceiving the patient into believing that his life is under threat. Again, the rough and violent treatments are meant to frighten the patient but never to seriously endanger him. Interestingly, just a few sentences before (Uttaratantra 62.12), Suśruta describes how the fear for one's life, but also the loss of what is dear to one, can be the very causes of madness.[452] Generally speaking, Suśruta's section on madness (*unmāda*) seems somewhat less structured than Caraka's treatment of the subject, which first gives the symptoms of each type of madness, followed by their remedies. While it is clear from Caraka's description that these particular fear-inducing treatments are meant for patients with *paittika* madness, this is not clearly categorized in the *Suśrutasaṃhitā*, indicating that these treatments may not have been fully understood in the latter tradition.

To conclude, in the ayurvedic classics, honesty is described as one of the qualities that define good conduct. For the medical authors, good conduct is not solely a matter of etiquette and social rules; it is part of a metaphysics that understands individual human behavior as having far-reaching consequences for the individual, for society, and for the environment at large. Bad conduct is seen as one of the root causes of illness and unhappiness in the individual, and it has similarly serious implications for human society as a whole. The medical classics offer clear categorizations of behaviors or actions as good or as bad, or rather as "to be done" or "not to be done," each respectively associated with health and happiness, or illness and misery. However, the classification of actions and behaviors does not necessarily translate into a moral characterization of the human beings displaying them. A certain tension is created by the medical authors between an idea of human beings as on the one hand creatures able to make moral decisions and to act on them and on the other as beings displaying tendencies to certain behaviors that are part of their nature. The former model makes humans active agents in a moral universe; the latter model places human action outside moral judgement. The question of how accountable human beings are for their actions remains somewhat unresolved by the medical authors, though the prevalent tendency displayed by them does seem to favor human agency. In fact, Caraka's admonition "one should not lie," as indeed all of the advice given in the medical texts' chapters on good conduct, only makes sense in the context of human agency. However, even if the premise of human agency with its potential for moral choice is accepted by the medical authors, their emphasis is never on abstract moral goals, but on the more tangible achievement of health and longevity.

Advice on good conduct in general is echoed by the medical authors' descriptions of desirable characteristics in a medical student. Several of the medical classics describe how in the medical student's initiation ceremony, the student is called on to be honest and to abandon untruth. This rule may pertain mainly to the student's behavior toward his teacher during his apprenticeship, but it is also described as a necessary behavior for the practicing physician "who wishes for success and wealth and the attainment of fame and heaven after death."[453]

Such advice is, however, contradicted, or at least somewhat reinterpreted, in the course of action proposed by Caraka in the case of a patient's imminent death. Here, he advises the physician not to tell the patient or his relatives the whole truth about the patient's condition if he considers it too upsetting for the patient. This introduces the first of the three contexts in which a physician's actions may break the general requirement of honesty, while remaining ethically correct. In the second context, physicians are advised to administer certain efficacious but disgusting meats disguised as more acceptable foods to patients. In the third context, deception is used to shock the patient into believing his life is at stake and thus to bring about the necessary changes in the patient's mental state. The role of dishonesty is different in each context. In the first, dishonesty is used to shield the patient from upsetting news. In the second, dishonesty is used to ensure patient compliance with the physician's prescription. In the third, deception is a central part of the therapeutic process: it is used as a medical tool, as it were. Each use of deception ultimately relies on the fundamental assumption that the physician has both a full understanding of the medical situation and bears the patient's best interests in mind. Thus, the doctor–patient relationship in Ayurveda is shown to be essentially paternalistic.

As a final observation, it needs to be pointed out that while the chosen excerpts from the medical texts display a certain amount of reference to the topic of honesty and deception in the doctor–patient relationship, the classical texts lack ethical metadiscussion of this topic entirely. Only the commentators—and particularly Caraka's commentator Cakrapāṇidatta—actually problematize the ethical dilemmas facing physicians in some of the situations depicted in the classics.

7

Ethical Elisions

THERE ARE A number of subjects one might expect in a study on medical ethics that have not been addressed in the preceding chapters. The main reason for this is that these are subject matters that find only little or even no mention in the classic ayurvedic treatises. They include topics such as violence in medicine, which encompasses such topical issues as abortion and euthanasia, but also the matter of violence that is inherent to standard medical practice (as for example, the use of painful therapies and of surgery).[454] Another important area of medical ethics surrounds the question of medical error and the related issues of responsibility and accountability. The scant or entirely lacking mention of such issues, which are now considered core areas of ethical questioning in medicine, is puzzling. However, the ayurvedic authors provide no pointers toward whether such topics were considered taboo or simply not worth mentioning. A brief overview follows of what can be found on these subjects in the classic ayurvedic treatises.

Violence

The topic of violence in medicine has been addressed in Francis Zimmermann's book *The Jungle and the Aroma of Meat*. Zimmermann explored the tension in the ayurvedic classics between a therapeutic system of purity, based on nonviolence, abstinence, and vegetarianism, and a therapeutic system of force and virility, in which there exists a certain amount of violence through the use of meat, purging, and so on. Zimmermann suggested that "the art of healing imposes the use of violence on the medical practitioner: violence towards animals if meats must be eaten, violence toward the patient if bloodletting, surgery, or obstetrics must be carried out."[455] However, Zimmermann saw no ethical dilemma for the physician in using violent therapies. Rather, he affirmed that "the use of violence degrades the position of medicine in the hierarchy of pure and impure activities, but in no way destroys its orthodoxy."[456] He also suggested that the conflicting elements of nonviolence and violence in medicine are reflections of the norms of two different social groups to which medicine caters: brahmins, members of the priest classes who espouse notions of purity and nonviolence, and the ruling classes (*kṣatriyas*), for whom the exercise of power (which may involve the use of violence) is their social function. Zimmermann discussed this dichotomy specifically in the context of the use of meat as part of a healthy diet and as part of medical therapy in order to explain why the use of meat appears not to be contentious in the ayurvedic treatises. The reason one would a priori expect the topic of meat consumption to be contentious is that the ayurvedic treatises align themselves in many instances with brahmanic norms. Proposing the use of meat, especially beef, seems to break with this alignment, since brahmanism is associated with vegetarianism, as well as with prohibitions concerning other foods that are also routinely recommended in the ayurvedic sources. Zimmermann (1999 [1987], 180–194), however, showed that there are instances in which the consumption of meat is normative behavior even for brahmins.[457]

It is important to note that we find no metadiscussion of violence that is inherent to standard medical practice in the Sanskrit medical classics.[458] We also find no indication of an awareness among the medical authors that giving a patient pain in order to achieve a positive therapeutic result could pose a moral dilemma to the physician. There are a number of occasions in which violence in general is stated to be a negative attribute,[459] while gentleness is praised as a positive characteristic of the physician.[460] Though the treatises mention the pain a patient experiences from an injury or an illness, the fact that some therapies, such as, for example, the cauterization of wounds, cause the patient pain is hardly acknowledged. Neither is the possibility discussed that a patient may experience fear of a potentially painful medical intervention.[461] In some special cases, both physical and psychological pain are used as a therapeutic tool to treat mentally ill patients (who are not aware that this is part of their therapy).[462] Again, there is no discussion of the moral implications of this therapeutic choice.

Abortion and Contraception

As regards abortion (in the sense of a deliberate effecting of a miscarriage), what little material can be found on the subject has been summarized by Julius Lipner in his essay "The Classical Hindu View on Abortion and the Moral Status of the Unborn." Describing Caraka's and Suśruta's views on ensoulment and consciousness in the womb, Lipner concludes that neither author proposes a moment of development in which the embryo undergoes "a quantum leap, passing from one kind of human moral status (human being) to another (human person)," that would allow for arguing for abortion.[463] Again, it should be noted that this discussion simply does not arise in these treatises. However, it is clear that abortions were known about and did take place, since Caraka mentions abortionists as persons whom a physician should strictly avoid.[464] In this, Caraka concurs with what was obviously a widely held view in his times: that the deliberate termination of a pregnancy was a reprehensible act. Discussing the moral evaluation of the act of abortion in some of the normative Hindu religious and religious law texts (Dharmasūtras and Dharmaśāstras, Purāṇas, and the epic Mahābhārata), Lipner (1989, 45) concludes that pregnancy was seen as "a very special state and that the unborn had a (moral) status meriting protection," while abortion was considered morally unacceptable and universally condemned.

While the act of abortion is generally not discussed in the classic medical treatises, there is one exception: In Su.Cik.15.11., Suśruta recommends that if an abnormality in a living fetus cannot be remedied at the time birth would normally take place, a miscarriage (*pātana*) should be caused in order to save the mother's life.[465] However, Suśruta does not provide a recipe for an abortive drug. In the context of how to remove a dead fetus, Caraka proposes that "some have said that the act of removal that causes the expulsion of the afterbirth is good for the extraction of the fetus."[466] Suśruta, however, does not make this connection, and clearly does not promote abortive practices.

In later medical works, we do encounter recipes for abortifacients, as well as for contraceptives, though no discussions of the ethics of their use. The earliest mention of recipes for contraceptives occurs in the *Bhāvaprakāśa* (Madhyakhaṇḍa 70 [*yonirogādhikāra*], 33–34), which gives two recipes:

> An embryo will never be produced by one who drinks Piper longum, Embelia ribes, and borax ground together with milk at the time of fertility.[467]

> A menstruating women who eats hibiscus blossom macerated in fermented rice gruel for three days together with a handful of old jaggery does not conceive.[468]

These recipes are found in between recipes for influencing the gender of the child to be born (i.e., ensuring that a male child will be born) and recipes for the treatment of vaginal diseases. Bhāvamiśra offers no further comments.

The first medical work that to my knowledge provides recipes for abortifacients is the *Yogacintāmaṇi*. Written in the late sixteenth or early seventeenth century by Harṣakīrti, a Jain monk resident in Nāgpur, this work devotes several verses to contraceptive measures and abortifacients.[469] The next work to provide such recipes is the *Vaidyavallabha* by Hastiruci, also a Jain monk, dated to about the late seventeenth century. The recipes for abortifacients occur in chapter 2, verses 18–23, and recipes for contraceptives are found in the same chapter in verses 26–31.[470] We find further recipes for both contraceptives and abortifacients in Trimallabhaṭṭa's *Yogataraṅginī* (chap. 75, verses 8–19), a work that is roughly dated to the seventeenth century. Its author was a brahmin.[471] There are also some abortifacient and contraceptive formulae in the late seventeenth-century *Vaidyarahasya* (in the chapter on disorders during pregnancy, verses 31–35) by Vidyāpati, a brahmin hailing from Mithilā.[472] Finally, the anonymous *Yogaratnākara*, tentatively dated to the late seventeenth or early eighteenth century, has a chapter on female diseases that also contains some recipes for abortifacients and contraceptives (verses 849–850).[473]

The recipes for contraceptives and abortifacients in the medical works are predated by formulae found in works that belong to a different literary genre: the *kāmaśāstra*, or "science of love." The *kāmaśāstra* tradition begins with Vātsyāyana's famous *Kāmasūtra* around the third century. However, the first work of this genre that gives recipes for abortifacients is the *Ratirahasya*, which was written by Kokokka in about the twelfth or thirteenth century.[474]

To summarize, recipes for contraceptives and abortifacients are first found in medical works in the sixteenth century and are predated by recipes found in the *Ratirashasya* by some three or four hundred years. Only a small number of medical works provides such recipes. It seems that none of these works offer any discussion of the ethical aspects of the use of contraceptives or abortifacients; they simply list recipes without any further commentary.

Euthanasia

The term "euthanasia" derives from the ancient Greek words for "good" (*eu-*) and "death" (*thanatos*) and in classical Greece referred to voluntary and self-imposed suicide, which could, however, be abetted, especially through the provision of poison.[475] While there is no universally accepted legal definition of "euthanasia" today, the term is usually used to describe compassionate killing in medically defined cases of terminal illness. Distinctions are made between voluntary (conducted with the informed consent of the patient), nonvoluntary (conducted where the consent of the patient is unavailable), and involuntary (conducted against the will of the patient) euthanasia. When the patient brings about his or her own death with the assistance of a physician, the term "assisted suicide" is often used instead. All types of euthanasia can be categorized as passive or active. Passive euthanasia entails the withholding of common treatments (for example, antibiotics) necessary for the continuance of life, while active euthanasia entails the use of lethal substances or forces to kill. The difference is, therefore, between letting die and killing.[476]

The ayurvedic classics yield no material on the topic of euthanasia either in the sense of self-willed death or of physician–assisted suicide. The idea that a patient might wish to die or to be let die (rather than having medical treatment) is not mentioned in any of the works, and we certainly find no directions on hastening a patient's death. The matter is simply not discussed in any way. The medical authors did have a great deal to say about dealing with terminally ill patients (as has been discussed in chapter 4). They generally advised physicians not to treat patients who were incurably ill and whose illnesses could not be managed. In other words, physicians were not to attempt treatment in cases where treatment would have been futile. Since the treatments would not have been necessary for the continuance of life, their withdrawal or withholding would not have constituted euthanasia. And indeed there is no hint in the ayurvedic classics that withdrawing treatment was seen as a way of expediting a patient's death.

Medical Error

One last topic that is not discussed in the main body of this study but deserves mention is medical error. In the medical treatises, medical error is described as something that happens only to a physician who is ignorant, or unskilled, that is, a quack. By definition (see chapter 1), a physician's well-considered actions are based on his profound knowledge of medicine and his extensively practiced skills. A good physician also chooses his patients carefully, avoiding those whose illnesses cannot be cured and those who would not comply with his prescriptions. In this scenario, medical error is not possible.[477]

On the other hand, from the large sections in the medical treatises dedicated to treating the results of mismanaged bloodletting or treatment with enemas, it is evident that things went wrong quite routinely in some kinds of treatment.[478] The lengthy and detailed descriptions of what may go wrong, how to avoid this, but also what to do if it happens nevertheless, pertain to risks any physician might expose the patient to in undertaking these treatments. However, the image of a perfect physician remains intact: treatments that go wrong are construed as being the work of ignorant or unskilled persons, while the good physician through his superior knowledge is in a position to undo the harm done by these quacks and to rescue the patient.[479]

8

Concluding Reflections

IN THE INTRODUCTION, the question was posed whether the classical ayurvedic treatises share basic ethical assumptions about good and bad medical practice that would allow us to speak not only of an ayurvedic ethic, but more specifically of an ayurvedic medical ethic: a set of moral values and rules that apply uniquely to the practice of medicine as opposed to human conduct in general.

To begin with, we can certainly state that while there are some divergences in detail and emphasis, the medical treatises share assumptions about good and bad or right and wrong behavior in medical practice. The treatises' prescriptions refer to all persons involved in a medical situation, but particularly focus on the physician. Their assumptions about correct conduct are given formalized expression in their definitions of the pillars of medicine and in the context of medical education. For example, Caraka integrates what amounts to a code of medical ethics into the initiation ceremony of the medical student. The other authors do not make their rules on professional conduct part of the initiation process itself but place them into context with it by positioning them in the same chapter. The *Suśrutasaṃhitā* is the exception to this: Suśruta devotes an entire separate chapter to the entry into the profession, the contents of which, however, are very similar to what the other authors propose.

The treatises' descriptions of a physician's good professional behavior are similar enough to each other to warrant the statement that the treatises share a common code of professional conduct—an ayurvedic medical ethic. However, this code of professional conduct is linked with a wider code of good conduct laid out by the medical authors in the context of healthy and virtuous living for all. Though the rules of good behavior for physicians and for everyone else are not a complete match, it seems that the good conduct of a physician was very similar to what would have been perceived as good conduct in general.

Furthermore, the ideas about good conduct proposed in the ayurvedic treatises do not represent a completely unique ayurvedic point of view: they have much in common with rules from brahmanic literature. As discussed, the medical student's initiation ceremony is strikingly similar to that of the

Vedic student and the rules of conduct for either student correspond in many details. In turn, the physician's code of conduct has strong similarities to rules of conduct for the Vedic bath-graduate. The ayurvedic rules of conduct for a good physician are only original in that they emphasize a particular kind of knowledge and skill. The more general rules of conduct echo those in brahmanic religious law literature and probably also reflect the dominant cultural conventions in the societies the medical authors lived in. By aligning their rules of conduct for the medical student with those for *brahmacārins*, the medical authors follow an established and accepted pattern of teacher–pupil interaction, presenting medical education as part of an orthodoxy. The rules of professional conduct are a continuation of this theme, as they present or represent medical practice as part of mainstream (brahmanic) cultural organization.

The formal expression of rules corresponding to understood rules and conventions of society positions the physician firmly within the in-group—the genteel parts of the society he lives in—and consequently lets him be perceived as safe. A physician needs to be both trust-inspiring and trust-deserving to be able to practice medicine for a living. His patients need not only to be safe in his hands but also to feel safe under his care. Being perceived as a member of the in-group makes a difference to a physician's acceptance in society. And according to the ayurvedic treatises, the physician's position was not only safely within the in-group but probably within its higher echelons. This mechanism of showing the physician to be part of mainstream (upper-class) society is, in my view, the function of the more formal codes of conduct found in the medical treatises.

However, the formalized expressions of the rules of good professional conduct shared by the treatises are juxtaposed with instances of less centrally positioned and sometimes also more implicitly phrased advice on conduct. It is in these instances that we sometimes see a divergence from brahmanic customs. This divergence is particularly notable in the area of the use of foods as medicinal substances. More often than not, the medical authors advise the use of foods that are prohibited in brahmanic law literature. The completely casual use of beef in the ayurvedic treatises is one example, the use of carnivores' meat another. In the context of the latter example, Caraka shows some awareness of the controversial nature of their use, which is entirely lacking in the context of the use of beef. His advice is to lie to the patients about the substances they are administered. This rather practical bit of advice relates not to the moral problem of serving problematic foods that have connotations of ritual impurity, but to the more direct problem of getting patients to eat something they feel disgusted by. This passage is remarkable in that it is one of the few instances in which a medical author actually gives a reason for proceeding in a particular way. While Caraka does not give any moral reasons for the actions he proposes, his commentator Cakrapāṇidatta picks up on another ethical conundrum: the question of a physician's duty to be honest, and how this may clash with Caraka's suggestion to lie to patients. Cakrapāṇidatta's conclusion on the matter is that there is no contradiction between the general rule that one should not lie (expressed in Ca.Sū.8.19) and the recommendation to disguise meats and offer them as other meats, "since the guilt of speaking falsehood is incurred by speaking untruth that results in harming another, but not by speaking untruly for the sake of another's life."[480]

This brings us to the question how the prescriptions of appropriate behavior found in the ayurvedic treatises relate to the concepts of ethics and morality. The medical treatises generally offer no metadiscussion of the moral implications of their prescriptions. They do not explain why any behavior should be considered right or wrong, only that it may be classified so. We find some metadiscussions in the commentaries, most notably in Cakrapāṇidatta's *Āyurvedadīpikā*. Even these, however, are scant. There is certainly no systematic philosophical study of the moral domain in which the medical authors seek to determine how moral outcomes can be achieved in specific situations or how moral values should be determined. Their presentation of the ethics of medical practice is mostly descriptive. We learn that a physician should do one thing, and must not do another. What is prescribed as good behavior is good in that it leads to a certain outcome. It is not clear whether the elements of good behavior represent an abstract value of goodness in themselves.

Caraka notes in the teacher's speech in Vi.8.13 that a physician should act in certain ways if he wishes for wealth, fame, and heaven after earth. These goals are the expected rewards of successful medical practice. To be successful, however, much is required of the physician. It is not enough that he have a thorough education that has equipped him with the requisite knowledge and skills, nor is it enough for him to follow the outer forms of etiquette in his behavior. He is required to live and practice according to an ethic that encompasses philanthropy and a wider concern for the happiness of all living beings, including a complete commitment to preserving or establishing the patient's welfare. Modesty and humility are an important part of his mental and emotional makeup. He must know for one thing that ayurvedic knowledge—the knowledge of life, no less!—is vast, and that he must constantly strive to perfect his knowledge and skills. He must also be aware, as Bhāvamiśra reminds us, that he is not the Lord of life: his power to help patients is limited by a number of factors.[481]

In the *Carakasaṃhitā* and in the *Aṣṭāṅgasaṃgraha* we find the virtues of loving kindness and compassion toward patients as a good physician's characteristics.[482] The phrasing of these terms shows a link to Buddhist thought (specifically to the Pāli Canon). Suśruta also proposes an emotional link between physician and patient that is based on benevolence on part of the physician and trust on part of the patient.[483] A similar statement is also found in the *Aṣṭāṅgasaṃgraha*.[484] The physician is urged to treat the patient like a son. This suggests that a physician should take great care in a patient's treatment, but also hints at a relationship based on love and responsibility. Suśruta argues that the physician must treat the patient as he would a son since the patient trusts him with his life. Being trusted, then, is what obliges the physician to be trustworthy, while the physician's attitude of love and care is what makes it possible for the patient to trust the physician. It should be noted, though, that the physician's obligation to treat a patient like his own child only pertains to those he accepts as patients. The medical authors all give instructions about persons a physician should not treat, whom he should avoid, and whom he should give up. It is particularly in the latter case that the ideals of kindness and compassion are put into question, since it is typically persons with terminal illnesses that a physician is meant to abandon. In other words, though he may have entered into the special father–child relationship with them, he will still give them up if he diagnoses them as incurable. The physician's decision to give up a patient would not be based on ill will or spite but on a realistic assessment of his ability to do anything against the illness and to alleviate the patient's suffering. Nevertheless, the suspicion remains that the abandonment of the patient serves the physician's needs rather than those of the patient.

While benevolent paternalism may have constituted the emotional background of medical interaction, it is not quite clear what form it took in the actual exchanges between physician and patient. There is, for example, hardly any description in the medical treatises of the physician speaking kind, calming, or consoling words to the patient, or of physical contact that isn't part of the treatment, such as holding the patient's hand.[485] There is mention of good friends providing such care in the *Carakasaṃhitā*.[486] However, the encounter between physician and patient mostly remains quite vague, even to a point where there is hardly a sense of any interaction between them. For example, if we look at Caraka's description of how the physician ought to behave in the patient's home, we do not find any description of his meeting with the patient. There is mention that the physician's attention should be fixed on the patient, but this is part of an admonition not to get tied up with the other people (most important, the women) in the patient's household. Most of the rules about how to act in the patient's home are about proper interaction with the other members of the house, and about respecting their privacy. A physician's confidentiality not only means keeping the patient's condition to himself, but also not gossiping about anything else he witnesses on his visit to someone's home. At a critical moment in the patient's care, when the physician has diagnosed the patient's imminent death, he does not relate this information to the patient (this possibility is not even raised) but to the relatives. This places communication with the patient at one remove (assuming that the relatives will in fact tell the patient of his approaching death).

There are, however, some instances in the *Carakasaṃhitā* in which the physician directly addresses the patient, giving him instructions on what to do in a therapeutic situation. One of the instances is described in Ca.Sū.14.46 in the context of admitting the patient to a kind of sauna room. There, the physician welcomes the patient to the sauna room and gives him instructions on where to lie down and how long to stay there. In another example (in Ca.Sū.15.12), the physician instructs the patient on what to do in the context of medicinally induced vomiting.

Suśruta describes some of the formal procedures of the therapeutic encounter between physician and patient. These begin with the summoning of the physician by a messenger. The arrival of the messenger is in some sense the first moment of diagnosis, since the way a messenger arrives is one of the signs that inform the physician about the patient's condition and the likelihood of his or her recovery. Finally, there is some description of contact between physician and patient: Having arrived at the patient's home, and having taken a seat, the physician "should have a good look at the patient, feel him, and question him."[487] A description of how to arrive at a diagnosis through the use of the senses (hearing, touch, sight, taste, and smell) and through asking questions follows. The patient is the physician's passive object of scrutiny. Only in the interrogation about his condition does he play an active part in the medical encounter. Giving exact and comprehensive information is one of the duties of the patient as laid out in the treatises' definitions of the pillars of treatment. This is more or less all we learn about the medical encounter between patient and physician.

We learn even less about the interactions between physicians and attendants. These are simply defined in terms of hierarchy, the physician being the superior of the attendant. The attendant is described as obedient to the physician. He is required to carry out the former's instructions, though the authors do not specify clearly what these instructions might be. There is some mention of preparing soups, and of massage, though this occurs in the specialized context of rejuvenative therapies that may have been only used for elite patients who were not actually ill. It is likely that the attendant took on the menial jobs of nursing, taking care of all the patient's needs who were not directly connected to medical intervention. However, these tasks may also have been taken on by the relatives of the patient. The attendant's relationship with the patient is thus a matter of some speculation. Midwives (as a subcategory of attendants) seem to have had a more independent position, perhaps even one of authority. They assisted at births, and this may have even been done without the presence of a physician, though the medical authors are not entirely clear on this point. In any case, according to the *Carakasaṃhitā*, the midwives' instructions at birth were regarded as authoritative and put on par with commands by brahmins officiating the rituals that accompanied the birth. The midwives' assistance at the birth also encompassed giving moral support and comforting the mother-to-be.

Last in the list of medical relationships stands the relationship between colleagues. There seems to have been quite a lot of competition between physicians, with strong claims being made for who was truly a physician and who was a quack. Some exchanges between physicians are described as benign and mutually beneficial. Kaśyapa puts forward the idea that physicians should prepare medicines together or in consultation with each other and admonishes physicians not to quarrel with each other. However, the guidance Kaśyapa gives on interaction between professionals is unique and finds no parallel in the other medical treatises. Several of the medical authors propose that physicians should engage in debate with each other as a method of enhancing their knowledge, but perhaps also as a way of marking out those whose knowledge might be deemed insufficient. According to Caraka (who gives the most information about quacks), one of the characteristics of a charlatan is that he will never discuss medical matters with peers. Another is that nothing is known of his medical provenance—from whom he learnt medicine. This indicates that physicians were familiar with other schools of thought (perhaps other teachers' special teachings) and were aware of other physicians, accepting some and rejecting others. The acceptance by other physicians would probably have been a matter of both belonging to an accepted group of physicians and having personal abilities and medical skills. Having undergone a formal initiation into medical studies, as described in most of the medical treatises, as well as having undertaken a period of study with an authoritative teacher may have formed the basis of other physicians' acceptance.

Last, I would like to turn to the question what the ultimate aims of medical practice were. According to Caraka, a physician's goals are to succeed in his practice, to accumulate wealth, to become famous, and finally, to reach heaven after death. At the same time, Caraka warns that physicians who practice only for money, "selling medical treatment as a trade, are devoted to a heap of dust, having abandoned gold."[488]

The meaning of practicing medicine is different for each class: It should be done "as a favor by brahmins, in order to protect by those of the governing classes, and for a livelihood by those of the trade classes, and generally by all of them to attain virtue, wealth, and pleasure."[489] Kaśyapa puts it even more strikingly:

> By brahmins for the sake of thorough knowledge, for their own merit, and in order to assist living beings, by those of the governing classes to protect their subjects, by those of the trade classes for a living, by the rest as service, and by all for the sake of virtue.[490]

This corresponds to a description in the *Manusmṛti* of the purpose of each class.[491] Practicing medicine in a particular way or with a particular aim thus can be understood to serve the purpose of fulfilling one's *dharma*, one's ethical role or purpose in life. The ethical practice of medicine according to the rules of one's class is thus part of moral living.

Caraka emphasizes that there is a virtue that surpasses all other considerations. He states that "one who practices medicine out of compassion toward all creatures rather than for wealth or pleasure overcomes all. . . . The practitioner of medicine who believes that his highest calling is the care of others achieves the highest happiness. He fulfills himself."[492]

This brings us back to the ayurvedic myth of the original transmission of ayurvedic knowledge to humans, in which a group of sages who were witnessing the decline in human health decided to seek help from the gods. The sages felt compassion for the plight of the other sentient beings. Their compassion was directed not only at the bodily discomforts caused by illness but also at the wider implications of disease as an impediment to virtuous living. Therefore, by learning about medicine, the sage-physicians in some sense meant to address moral as well as physical ills. This may be what the medical authors envisaged as any physician's goals: alleviating suffering and providing health as the foundation for a virtuous life.

Cakrapāṇidatta (*on* Ca.Sū.8.29) claims that "the rules of ayurveda do not teach the achievement of righteousness. Rather, they teach the achievement of health."[493] This may be true in the first instance, and certainly explains those rules in the treatises that run counter to brahmanic rules. There is a paradox here: The goal of achieving the cure of a patient may lead to actions that seem to go against brahmanic rules of behavior. However, by doing all he can to cure the patient the physician may be understood to be acting according to his specific *dharma* as a physician. This would mean that his actions are ethically correct and fit in with brahmanic orthodoxy. The medical authors thus may not propose the achievement of righteousness as an immediate goal, but still understand righteousness to be central to medical practice.

APPENDICES

Sanskrit Text Passages

APPENDIX A

The Pillars of Treatment

Definitions of the Pillars of Treatment

The Four Pillars of Treatment According to Caraka

Carakasaṃhitā Sūtrasthāna 9

navamo 'dhyāyaḥ |
athātaḥ khuḍḍākacatuṣpādam adhyāyaṃ vyākhyāsyāmaḥ ||1||
iti ha smāha bhagavān ātreyaḥ[494] ||2||
bhiṣag dravyāṇy upasthātā rogī pādacatuṣṭayam |
guṇavat kāraṇaṃ jñeyaṃ vikāravyupaśāntaye ||3||
vikāro dhātuvaiṣamyaṃ sāmyaṃ prakṛtir ucyate |
sukhasaṃjñakam ārogyaṃ vikāro duḥkham eva ca ||4||
caturṇāṃ bhiṣagādīnāṃ śastānāṃ dhātuvaikṛte |
pravṛttir dhātusāmyārthā cikitsety abhidhīyate ||5||
śrute paryavadātatvaṃ bahuśo dṛṣṭakarmatā |
dākṣyaṃ śaucam iti jñeyaṃ vaidye guṇacatuṣṭayam ||6||
bahutā tatrayogyatvam anekavidhakalpanā |
saṃpac ceti catuṣko 'yaṃ dravyāṇāṃ guṇa ucyate ||7||
upacārajñatā dākṣyam anurāgaś ca bhartari |
śaucaṃ ceti catuṣko 'yaṃ guṇaḥ paricare jane ||8||
smṛtir nirdeśakāritvam abhīrutvam athāpi ca |
jñāpakatvaṃ ca rogāṇām āturasya guṇāḥ smṛtāḥ ||9||
kāraṇaṃ ṣoḍaśaguṇaṃ siddhau pādacatuṣṭayam |
vijñātā śāsitā yoktā pradhānaṃ bhiṣag atra tu ||10||
paktau hi kāraṇaṃ paktur yathā pātrendhanānalāḥ |
vijetur vijaye bhūmiś camūḥ praharaṇāni ca ||11||
āturādyās tathā siddhau pādāḥ kāraṇasaṃjñitāḥ |
vaidyasya ataś cikitsāyāṃ pradhānaṃ kāraṇaṃ bhiṣak ||12||
mṛddaṇḍacakrasūtrādyāḥ kumbhakārād ṛte yathā |
nāvahanti guṇaṃ vaidyād ṛte pādatrayaṃ tathā ||13||
gandharvapuravan nāśaṃ yad vikārāḥ sudāruṇāḥ |
yānti yac cetare vṛddhim āśūpāyapratīkṣiṇaḥ ||14||
sati pādatraye jñājñau bhiṣajāv atra kāraṇam |
varam ātmā huto 'jñena na cikitsā pravartitā ||15||

pāṇicārād yathācakṣur ajñānād bhītabhītavat|
naur mārutavaśevājño bhiṣak carati karmasu ||16||
yadṛcchayā samāpannam uttārya niyatāyuṣam |
bhiṣaṅmānī nihanty āśu śatāny aniyatāyuṣām ||17||
tasmāc chāstre 'rthavijñāne pravṛttau karmadarśane|
bhiṣak catuṣṭaye yuktaḥ prāṇābhisara ucyate ||18||
hetau liṅge praśamane rogāṇām apunarbhave |
jñānaṃ caturvidhaṃ yasya sa rājārho bhiṣaktamaḥ ||19||
śastraṃ śāstrāṇi salilaṃ guṇadoṣapravṛttaye |
pātrāpekṣīṇy ataḥ prajñāṃ cikitsārthaṃ viśodhayet ||20||
vidyā vitarko vijñānaṃ smṛtis tatparatā kriyā |
yasyaite ṣaḍ guṇās tasya na sādhyam ativartate ||21||
vidyā matiḥ karmadṛṣṭir abhyāsaḥ siddhir āśrayaḥ |
vaidyaśabdābhiniṣpattāv alam ekaikam apy ataḥ ||22||
yasya tv ete guṇāḥ sarve santi vidyādayaḥ śubhāḥ |
sa vaidyaśabdaṃ sadbhūtam arhan prāṇisukhapradaḥ ||23||
śāstraṃ jyotiḥ prakāśārthaṃ darśanaṃ buddhir ātmanaḥ |
tābhyāṃ bhiṣak suyuktābhyāṃ cikitsan nāparādhyati ||24||
cikitsate trayaḥ pādā yasmād vaidyavyapāśrayaḥ |
tasmāt prayatnam ātiṣṭhed bhiṣak svaguṇasaṃpadi ||25||
maitrī kāruṇyam ārteṣu śakye prītir upekṣaṇam |
prakṛtistheṣu bhūteṣu vaidyavṛttiś caturvidheti ||26||

The Four Pillars of Treatment According to Suśruta

Suśrutasaṃhitā Sūtrasthāna 34.15cd–24

vaidyo vyādhyupasṛṣṭaś ca bheṣajaṃ paricārakaḥ ||15cd||
ete pādāś cikitsāyāḥ karmasādhanahetavaḥ ||
guṇavadbhis tribhiḥ pādaiś caturtho guṇavān bhiṣak ||16||
vyādhim alpena kālena mahāntam api sādhayet ||
vaidyahīnās trayaḥ pādā guṇavanto 'py apārthakāḥ ||17||
udgātṛhotṛbrahmāṇo yathādhvaryuṃ vinādhvare ||
vaidyas tu guṇavān ekas tārayed āturaṃ sadā ||18||
plavaṃ pratitarair hīnaṃ karṇadhāra ivāmbhasi ||
tattvādhigataśāstrārtho dṛṣṭakarmā svayaṃkṛtī ||19||
laghuhastaḥ śuciḥ śūraḥ sajjopaskarabheṣajaḥ ||
pratyutpannamatir dhīmān vyavasāyī viśāradaḥ ||20||
satyadharmaparo yaś ca sa bhiṣak pāda ucyate ||
āyuṣmān sattvavān sādhyo dravyavān ātmavān api ||21||
āstiko vaidyavākyastho vyādhitaḥ pāda ucyate ||
praśastadeśasaṃbhūtaṃ praśaste 'hani coddhṛtam ||22||
yuktamātraṃ manaskāntaṃ gandhavarṇarasānvitam ||

doṣaghnam aglānikaram avikāri viparyaye ||
samīkṣya dattaṃ kāle ca bheṣajaṃ pāda ucyate ||23||
snigdho 'jugupsur balavān yukto vyādhitarakṣaṇe ||
vaidyavākyakṛd aśrāntaḥ pādaḥ paricaraḥ smṛtaḥ ||24||

The Four Pillars of Treatment According to Vāgbhaṭa

Aṣṭāṅgahṛdayasaṃhitā Sūtrasthāna 1.27–29 and *Aṣṭāṅgasaṃgraha Sūtrasthāna 2.21–25ab*

bhiṣak dravyāṇy upasthātā rogī pādacatuṣṭayam |
cikitsitasya nirdiṣṭaṃ pratyekaṃ tac caturguṇam ||27||
dakṣas tīrthāttaśāstrārtho dṛṣṭakarmā śucir bhiṣak |
bahukalpaṃ bahuguṇaṃ sampannaṃ yogyam auṣadham ||28||
anuraktaḥ śucir dakṣo buddhimān paricārakaḥ |
āḍhyo rogī bhiṣagvaśyo jñāpakaḥ sattvavān api ||29||

The Four Pillars of Treatment According to Kaśyapa

Kāśyapasaṃhitā Sūtrasthāna 26.3–11

cikitsāsaṃpad yathopapadyate tamupāyam anuvyākhyāsyāmaḥ|
catvāraḥ khalu pādāś cikitsitasyopapadyante |
te yadā guṇavanta upapadyante tadā sādhyo vyādhir nātivartate |
tadyathā bhiṣak bheṣajam āturaḥ paricāraka iti ||3||
tatra bhiṣak sutīrtho nyāyenārṣajñānaprāpto vijñānavān anekaśo dṛṣṭakarmā viditasiddhayogo dakṣo dakṣiṇaḥ śucir anuddhataveṣaḥ sarvabhūteṣu bandhubhūtaḥ siddhimān dharmārthadarśī satyadayādānārjavanirato devadvijagurusiddhānāṃ pūjayitā cābhigantā cottarottarapratipattikuṣalo guruvṛddhasevī nyāyābhiniveṣī vyapagatabhayalobhamohakrodhānṛto 'paiṣunyo 'madyalaulyaḥ sumukhaś cāvyasanī ceti ||4||
tatra bheṣajasaṃpat subhūmau jātaṃ kāle coddhṛtaṃ kāle cotpannam avikāri agnitoyajantuviṇmūtrajarādibhir anupahataṃ tattadrogayogyaṃ krameṇa ca vidhivad upapāditam iti ||5||
tatrāturasaṃpat sādhyarogatā tattvabalabuddhiśarīrendriyadhṛtitejasāṃ dārḍhyaṃ, nidānapūrvarūpātaṅkopadravayātropaśayānupaśayānāṃ yathāvadākhyānaṃ dhātryā vā śraddadhānatā devadvijagurubhiṣagbheṣajasuhṛdām abhinandanam āstikyaṃ vinayapradhānatā yathoktakāritvaṃ vaśitvaṃ ceti ||6||
tatra paricārakasaṃpat—vipakvakaṣāyatā ārogyaṃ śaktiḥ bhartṛbhaktiḥ upacārajñatā dākṣkyaṃ śaucam āśukāritvaṃ sarvakarmasu kauśalam aghṛṇitvam akṣudraputratvam advaividhyaṃ damo jitakrodhāditā sahiṣṇutā ceti ||7||
tatra ślokāḥ |
asya pādacatuṣkasya manyante śreṣṭham āturam |
tadarthaṃ guṇavanto hi trayaḥ pādā ihepsitāḥ ||8||

neti prajāpatiḥ prāha bhiṣaṅ mūlaṃ cikitsitam |
bhiṣagvaśe trivargo hi siddhiś ca bhiṣaji sthitā ||9||
sa yunakti prajuṅkte ca śāsti ca jñānacakṣuṣā |
tasmāj jñāne savijñāne yuktaḥ śreṣṭhamo bhiṣak ||10||
yadā caturṇāṃ pādānāṃ saṃpad bhavati jīvaka |
tadā dharmārthayaśasāṃ vaidyo bhavati bhājanam ||11||

The Components of Treatment According to Bhāvamiśra

Bhāvaprakāśa Pūrvakhaṇḍa 6.37–54

atha cikitsāyā aṅgāny āha—
rogī dūto bhiṣag dīrgham āyur dravyaṃ susevakaḥ |
sadauṣadhaṃ cikitsāyā ity aṅgāni budhā jaguḥ ||37||
tatra rogiṇo lakṣaṇam āha—
rogo yasyāsti rogī sa, sa[495] cikitsyas tu yādṛśaḥ |
yādṛśaś cācikitsyo 'pi vakṣyamāṇo niśamyatām ||38||
tatra cikitsyasya lakṣaṇam āha—
nijaprakṛtivarṇābhyāṃ yuktaḥ sattvena cakṣuṣā |
cikitsyo bhiṣajāṃ rogī vaidyabhakto jitendriyaḥ ||39||[496]
anyac ca āyuṣmān sattvavān sādhyo dravyavān mitravān api |
cikitsyo bhiṣajāṃ rogī vaidyavākyakṛd āstikaḥ ||40||[497]
athācikitsyasya lakṣaṇam āha—
caṇḍaḥ sāhasiko bhīruḥ kṛtaghno vyagra eva ca |
śokākulo mumūrṣuś ca vihīnaḥ karaṇaiś ca yaḥ ||41||
vairī vaidyavidagdhaś ca śraddhāhīnaś ca śaṅkitaḥ |
bhiṣajām avidheyaḥ syur nopakramyā bhiṣagvidāḥ[498] ||42||
athācikitsyānāṃ cikitsāniṣedham āha—
etān upācaran vaidyo bahūn doṣān avāpnuyāt ||43||
atha dūtasya lakṣaṇam āha—
yaś cikitsakam ānetuṃ yāti dūtaḥ sa kathyate |
sa ca yādṛk samucitas tādṛg atra nigadyate ||44||
dūtāḥ sujātayo 'vyaṅgāḥ paṭavo nirmalāmbarāḥ |
sukhino 'śvavṛṣārūḍhāḥ śubhrapuṣpaphalair yutāḥ ||45||
sajātayaḥ suceṣṭāś ca sajīvadiśi saṅgatāḥ |
bhiṣajaṃ samaye prāptā rogiṇaḥ sukhahetave ||46||[499]
atha dūtasya yātrāyāṃ śakunavicāram āha—
vaidyāhvānāya dūtasya gacchato rogiṇaḥ kṛte |
na śubhaṃ saumyaśakunaṃ pradīptaṃ tu sukhāvaham ||47||
atha dūto rogī ca riktahasto vaidyaṃ na paśyed ity āha—
tathāhi riktahasto na paśyet tu rājānaṃ bhiṣajaṃ gurum |
daivajñaṃ devatāṃ mitraṃ phalena phalam ādiśet ||48||
atha suvaidyasya lakṣaṇam āha—

cikitsāṃ kurute yas tu sa cikitsaka ucyate |
sa ca yādṛk samīcīnas tādṛśo 'pi nigadyate | |49| |
tattvādhigataśāstrārtho dṛṣṭakarmā svayaṃkṛtī |
laghuhastaḥ śuciḥ śūraḥ sajjopaskarabheṣajaḥ | |50| |
pratyutpannamatir dhīmān vyavasāyī priyaṃvadaḥ |
satyadharmaparo yaś ca vaidya īdṛk praśasyate[500] | |51| |
atha niṣiddhavaidyasya lakṣaṇam āha—
kucailaḥ karkaśaḥ stabdho grāmīṇaḥ svayam āgataḥ |
pañca vaidyā na pūjyante dhanvantarisamā yadi | |52| |
atha vaidyasya karmāha—
vyādhes tattvaparijñānaṃ vedanāyāś ca nigrahaḥ |
etad vaidyasya vaidyatvaṃ na vaidyaḥ prabhur āyuṣaḥ | |53| |
athāyurvicāram āha—
bhiṣag ādau parīkṣeta rugṇasyāyuḥ prayatnataḥ |
tata āyuṣi vistīrṇe cikitsā saphalā bhavet | |54| |

Bhāvaprakāśa Pūrvakhaṇḍa 6.88–92

atha dravyāvaśyakatām āha—
sarve dravyam apekṣante rogiprabhṛtayo yataḥ |
vinā vittaṃ na bhaiṣajyaṃ cikitsāṅgaṃ tato dhanam | |88| |
atha paricārakasya lakṣaṇam āha—
snigdho 'jugupsur balavān yukto vyādhitarakṣaṇe |
vaidyavākyakṛd aśrānto yujyate paricārakaḥ | |89| |[501]
atha bheṣajasya lakṣaṇam āha—
vaidyo vyādhiṃ hared yena tad dravyaṃ proktam auṣadham |
tad yādṛśam avaśyaṃ syād rogaghnaṃ tādṛśaṃ bruve | |90| |
athauṣadhagrahaṇaparibhāṣām āha—
praśastadeśe sañjātaṃ praśaste 'hani coddhṛtam |
alpamātraṃ bahuguṇaṃ gandhavarṇarasānvitam | |91| |
doṣaghnam aglānikaram adhikaṃ na vikāri yat |
samīkṣya kāle dattaṃ ca bheṣajaṃ syād guṇāvaham | |92| |[502]

The Physician, the Patient, and the Attendant

The Physician

Carakasaṃhitā Vimānasthāna 8.86

bhiṣaṅ nāma yo bhiṣajyati, yaḥ sūtrārthaprayogakuśalaḥ yasya cāyuḥ sarvathā viditaṃ yathāvat sa ca sarvadhātusāmyaṃ cikīrṣann ātmānam evāditaḥ parīkṣeta | guṇiṣu guṇataḥ kāryābhinirvṛttiṃ paśyan kaccid aham asya kāryasyābhinirvartane samartho na veti, tatreme bhiṣagguṇā yair upapanno bhiṣag dhātusāmyābhinirvartane samartho bhavati tadyathā – paryavadātaśrutatā paridṛṣṭakarmatā dākṣyaṃ śaucaṃ jitahastatā upakaraṇavattā sarvendriyopapannatā prakṛtijñatā pratipattijñatā ceti ||86||

Suśrutasaṃhitā Sūtrasthāna 3.48–50, 52

yas tu kevalaśāstrajñaḥ karmasv aparinișṭhitaḥ |
sa muhyaty āturaṃ prāpya prāpya bhīrur ivāhavam ||48||
yas tu karmasu niṣṇāto dhārṣṭyāc chāstrabahiṣkṛtaḥ |
sa satsu pūjāṃ nāpnoti vadhaṃ carcchati rājataḥ ||49||
ubhāv etāv anipuṇāv asamarthau svakarmaṇi |
ardhavedadharāv etāv ekapakṣāv iva dvijau ||50||
(. . .)
snehādiṣv anabhijño yaś chedyādiṣu ca karmasu |
sa nihanti janaṃ lobhāt kuvaidyo nṛpadoṣataḥ ||52||

Suśrutasaṃhitā Sūtrasthāna 4.7–8

śāstraṃ gurumukhodgīrṇam ādāyopāsya cāsakṛt |
yaḥ karma kurute vaidyaḥ sa vaidyo 'nye tu taskarāḥ ||8||

Carakasaṃhitā Sūtrasthāna 11.50–53

trividhā bhiṣaja iti—
bhiṣakchadmacarāḥ santi santy eke siddhasādhitāḥ |
santi vaidyaguṇair yuktās trividhā bhiṣajo bhuvi ||50||
vaidyabhāṇḍauṣadhaiḥ pustaiḥ pallavair avalokanaiḥ |
labhante ye bhiṣakśabdam ajñās te pratirūpakāḥ ||51||
śrīyaśojñānasiddhānāṃ vyapadeśād atadvidhāḥ |
vaidyaśabdaṃ labhante ye jñeyās te siddhasādhitāḥ ||52||
prayogajñānavijñānasiddhisiddhāḥ sukhapradāḥ |
jīvitābhisarās te syur vaidyatvaṃ teṣv avasthitam ||53||

Carakasaṃhitā Sūtrasthāna 29.4, 5, and 7 (first and last paragraph)

tānīndriyāṇi vijñānaṃ cetanāhetum āmayān |
jānīte yaḥ sa vai vidvān prāṇābhisara ucyate ||4||
dvividhās tu khalu bhiṣajo bhavanty agniveśa |
prāṇānām eke 'bhisarā hantāro rogāṇāṃ rogāṇām eke 'bhisarā hantāraḥ prāṇānām iti ||5||
(. . .)
ya ime kulīnāḥ paryavadātaśrutāḥ paridṛṣṭakarmāṇo dakṣāḥ śucayo jitahastā jitātmānaḥ sarvopakaraṇavantaḥ sarvendriyopapannāḥ prakṛtijñāḥ pratipattijñāś ca te jñeyāḥ prāṇānām abhisarā hantāro rogāṇāṃ,
(. . .)

kuśalāś ca smṛtimatiśāstrayuktijñānasyātmanaḥ śīlaguṇair avisaṃvādanena ca saṃpādanena sarvaprāṇiṣu cetaso maitrasya mātāpitṛbhrātṛbandhuvat evaṃyuktā bhavanty agniveśa | prāṇānām abhisarā hantāro rogāṇām iti||7||

Suśrutasaṃhitā Sūtrasthāna 25.41

ātmānam evātha jaghanyakārī śastreṇa yo hanti hi karma kurvan | tam ātmavān ātmahanaṃ kuvaidyaṃ vivarjayed āyurabhīpsamānaḥ ||41||

Suśrutasaṃhitā Sūtrasthāna 25.32

taṃ kṣāraśastrāgnibhir auṣadhaiś ca bhūyo 'bhiyuñjānam ayuktiyuktam | jijīviṣur dūrata eva vaidyaṃ vivarjayed ugraviṣāhitulyam ||32||

Carakasaṃhitā Sūtrasthāna 1.126–131, 135

yogād api viṣaṃ tīkṣṇam uttamaṃ bheṣajaṃ bhavet |
bheṣajaṃ cāpi duryuktaṃ tīkṣṇaṃ saṃpadyate viṣam ||126||
tasmān na bhiṣajā yuktaṃ yuktibāhyena bheṣajam |
dhīmatā kiṃcid ādeyaṃ jīvitārogyakāṅkṣiṇā ||127||
kuryān nipatito mūrdhni saśeṣaṃ vāsavāśaniḥ |
saśeṣam āturaṃ kuryān na tv ajñamatam auṣadham ||128||
duḥkhitāya śayānāya śraddadhānāya rogiṇe |
yo bheṣajam avijñāya prājñamānī prayacchati ||129||
tyaktadharmasya pāpasya mṛtyubhūtasya durmateḥ |
naro narakapātī syāt tasya saṃbhāṣaṇād api ||130||
varam āśīviṣaviṣaṃ kvathitaṃ tāmram eva vā |
pītam atyagnisantaptā bhakṣitā vāpy ayoguḍāḥ ||131||
(. . .)
samyakprayogaṃ sarveṣāṃ siddhir ākhyāti karmaṇām |
siddhir ākhyāti sarvaiś ca guṇair yuktaṃ bhiṣaktamam ||135||

Carakasaṃhitā Sūtrasthāna 29.8–9

ato viparītā rogāṇām abhisarā hantāraḥ prāṇānāṃ bhiṣakchadmapraticchannāḥ kaṇṭakabhūtā lokasya pratirūpakas adharmāṇo rājñāṃ pramādāc caranti rāṣṭrāṇi ||8|| teṣām idaṃ viśeṣavijñānaṃ bhavati atyarthaṃ vaidyaveśena ślāghamānā viśikhāntaram anucaranti karmalobhāt śrutvā ca kasyacid āturyam abhitaḥ paripatanti saṃśravaṇe cāsyātmano vaidyaguṇānudyair vadanti yaś cāsya vaidyaḥ pratikarma karoti tasya ca doṣān muhurmuhur udāharanti āturam itrāṇi ca praharṣaṇopajāpopasevādibhir icchanty ātmīkartuṃ svalpecchutāṃ cātmanaḥ khyāpayanti karma cāsādya muhurmuhur avalokayanti dākṣyeṇājñānam ātmanaḥ pracchādayitukāmāḥ vyādhiṃ cāpāvartayitum aśaknuvato vyādhitam evānupakaraṇam aparicārakam anātmavantam upadiśanti
antagataṃ cainam abhisamīkṣyānyam āśrayanti deśam apadeśam ātmanaḥ kṛtvā prākṛtajanasannipāte cātmanaḥ kauśalam akuśalavad varṇayanti adhīravac ca dhairyam apavadanti dhīrāṇāṃ vidvajjanasannipātaṃ cābhisamīkṣya pratibhayam

iva kāntāram adhvagāḥ pariharanti dūrāt yaś caiṣāṃ kaścit sūtrāvayavo bhavaty upayuktas tam aprakṛte prakṛtāntare vā satatam udāharanti na cānuyogam icchanty anuyoktuṃ vā mṛtyor iva cānuyogād udvijante na caiṣām ācāryaḥ śiṣyaḥ sabrahmacārī vaivādiko vā kaścit prajñāyata iti ||9||

The Patient

Carakasaṃhitā Siddhisthāna 11.27–30

athāgniveśaḥ satatāturān narān hitaṃ ca papraccha gurus tadāha ca |
sadāturāḥ śrotriyarājasevakās tathaiva veśyā saha paṇyajīvibhiḥ ||27||
dvijo hi vedādhyayanavratāhnikakriyādibhir dehahitaṃ na ceṣṭate |
nṛpopasevī nṛpacittarakṣaṇāt parānurodhād bahucintanād bhayāt ||28||
nṛcittavartiny upacāratatparā mṛjābhibhūṣāniratā paṇāṅganā |
sadāsanād atyanubandhavikrayakrayādilobhād api paṇyajīvinaḥ ||29||
sadaiva te hy āgataveganigrahaṃ samācarante na ca kālabhojanam |
akālanirhāravihārasevino bhavanti ye 'nye 'pi sadāturāś ca te ||30||

Aṣṭāṅgahṛdayasaṃhitā Śārīrasthāna 6.71cd–73ab

maṅgalācārasampannaḥ parivāras tathāturaḥ ||71||
śraddadhāno 'nukūlaś ca prabhūtadravyasaṅgrahaḥ |
sattvalakṣaṇasaṃyogo bhaktir vaidyadvijātiṣu ||72||
cikitsāyām anirvedas tad ārogyasya lakṣaṇam |

Suśrutasaṃhitā Sūtrasthāna 2.8

dvijagurudaridramitrapravrajitopanatasādhvanāthābhyupagatānāṃ cātmabāndhavānām iva svabhaiṣajaiḥ pratikartavyam, evaṃ sādhu bhavati, vyādhaśākunikapatitapāpakāriṇāṃ ca na pratikartavyam, evaṃ vidyā prakāśate mitrayaśodharmārthakāmāṃś ca prāpnoti ||8||

Suśrutasaṃhitā Sūtrasthāna 10.8

tatra sādhyā api vyādhayaḥ prāyeṇaiṣāṃ duścikitsyatamā bhavanti; tadyathā—śrotriyanṛpatistrībālavṛddhabhīrurājasevakakitavadurbalavaidyavidagdhavyādhigopakadaridrakṛpaṇakrodhanānām anātmavatām anāthānāṃ ca; evaṃ nirūpya cikitsāṃ kurvan dharmārthakāmayaśāṃsi prāpnoti ||8||

Suśrutasaṃhitā Sūtrasthāna 34.10cd–12ab

puruṣāṇāṃ nṛpāṇāṃ ca kevalaṃ tulyamūrtitā ||10||
ājñā tyāgaḥ kṣamā dhairyaṃ vikramaś cāpy amānuṣaḥ ||
tasmād devam ivābhīkṣṇaṃ vāṅmanaḥkarmabhiḥ śubhaiḥ ||11||
cintayen nṛpatiṃ vaidyaḥ śreyāṃsīcchan vicakṣaṇaḥ ||

Carakasaṃhitā Vimānasthāna 3.45–46

anapavādapratīkārasyādhanasyāparicārakasya vaidyamāninaś caṇḍasyāsūyakasya tīvrādharmarucer[503] atikṣīṇabalamāṃsaśoṇitasyāsādhyarogopahatasya mumūrṣu-

liṅgānvitasya ceti | evaṃvidhaṃ hy āturam upacaran bhiṣak pāpīyasāyaśasā yogam ṛcchatīti ||45||
bhavati cātra—
tadātve cānubandhe vā yasya syād aśubhaṃ phalam |
karmaṇas tan na kartavyam etad buddhimatāṃ matam ||46||

Carakasaṃhitā Siddhisthāna 2.4–6

caṇḍaḥ sāhasiko bhīruḥ kṛtaghno vyagra eva ca |
sadrājabhiṣajāṃ dveṣṭā taddviṣṭaḥ śokapīḍitaḥ ||4||
yādṛcchiko mumūrṣuś ca vihīnaḥ karaṇaiś ca yaḥ |
vairī vaidyavidagdhaś ca śraddhāhīnaḥ suśaṅkitaḥ ||5||
bhiṣajām avidheyaś ca nopakramyā bhiṣagvidā |
etān upacaran vaidyo bahūn doṣān avāpnuyāt ||6||

Aṣṭāṅgahṛdayasaṃhitā Sūtrasthāna 1.34–35ab

tyajed ārtaṃ bhiṣag bhūpair dviṣṭaṃ teṣāṃ dviṣaṃ dviṣam |
hīnopakaraṇaṃ vyagram avidheyaṃ gatāyuṣam ||34||
caṇḍaṃ śokāturaṃ bhīruṃ kṛtaghnaṃ vaidyamāninam|

Suśrutasaṃhitā Cikitsāsthāna 24.90

na rājadviṣṭaparuṣapaiśunyānṛtāni vadet, na devabrāhmaṇapitṛparivādāṃś ca, na narendradviṣṭonmattapatitakṣudranīcān upāsīta ||90||

Carakasaṃhitā Sūtrasthāna 8.19 (middle part)

nādhārmikair na narendradviṣṭaiḥ sahāsīta nonmattair na patitair na bhrūṇahantṛbhir na kṣudrair na duṣṭaiḥ

The Attendant and Other Helpers

Suśrutasaṃhitā Kalpasthāna 1.8–11

kulīnaṃ dhārmikaṃ snigdhaṃ subhṛtaṃ saṃtatotthitam |
alubdham aśaṭhaṃ bhaktaṃ kṛtajñaṃ priyadarśanam ||8||
krodhapāruṣyamātsaryamāyālasya vivarjitam |
jitendriyaṃ kṣamāvantaṃ śuciṃ śīladayānvitam ||9||
medhāvinam asaṃśrāntam anuraktaṃ hitaiṣiṇam |
paṭuṃ pragalbhaṃ nipuṇaṃ dakṣam ālasyavarjitam ||10||
pūrvoktaiś ca guṇair yuktaṃ nityaṃ sannihitāgadam |
mahānase prayuñjīta vaidyaṃ tadvidyapūjitam ||11||

Carakasaṃhitā Sūtrasthāna 15.7 (first part)

tataḥśīlaśaucācārānurāgadākṣyaprādakṣiṇyopapannānupacārakuśalān sarvakarmasu paryavadātān sūpaudanapācakasnāpakasaṃvāhakotthāpakasaṃveśakauṣadhapeṣakāṃś ca paricārakān sarvakarmasvapratikūlān tathā gītavāditrollāpakaślokagāthākhyāyiketihāsapurāṇakuśalān abhiprāyajñānanumatāṃś ca deśakālavidaḥ pāriṣadyāṃś ca

Carakasaṃhitā Sūtrasthāna 15.7 (last part)

yac cānyad api kiñcid vyāpadaḥ parisaṃkhyāya pratīkārārtham upakaraṇaṃ vidyāt, yac ca pratibhogārthaṃ, tat tad upakalpayet ||7||

Kitchen Staff

Suśrutasaṃhitā Kalpasthāna 1.13cd–18ab

parīkṣitastrīpuruṣaṃ bhavec cāpi mahānasam ||13||
tatrādhyakṣaṃ niyuñjīta prāyo vaidyaguṇānvitam |
śucayo dakṣiṇā dakṣā vinītāḥ priyadarśanāḥ ||14||
saṃvibhaktāḥ sumanaso nīcakeśanakhāḥ sthirāḥ |
snātā dṛḍhaṃ saṃyaminaḥ kṛtoṣṇīṣāḥ susaṃyatāḥ ||15||
tasya cājñāvidheyāḥ syur vividhāḥ parikarmiṇaḥ |
āhārasthitayaś cāpi bhavanti prāṇino yataḥ ||16||
tasmān mahānase vaidyaḥ pramādarahito bhavet||
māhānasikavoḍhāraḥ saupaudanikapaupikāḥ ||17||
bhaveyur vaidyavaśagā ye cāpy anye 'tra kecana||

Friends

Carakasaṃhitā Sūtrasthāna 5.11 (last part)

lālāṭapratigrahe pārśvopagrahaṇe nābhiprapīḍane pṛṣṭhonmardane cānapatrapaṇīyāḥ suhṛdo 'numatāḥ prayateran ||11||

Midwives and Experienced Women

Carakasaṃhitā Śārīrasthāna 8.34, 37

striyaś ca bahvyo bahuśaḥ prajātāḥ sauhārdayuktāḥ satatam anuraktāḥ pradakṣiṇācārāḥ pratipattikuśalāḥ prakṛtivatsalās tyaktaviṣādāḥ kleśasahinyo 'bhimatāḥ, brāhmaṇāś cātharvavedavidaḥ yac cānyad api tatra samarthaṃ manyeta yac cānyac ca brāhmaṇā brūyuḥ striyaś ca vṛdhās tat kāryam ||34||

(...)

āvīprādurbhāve tu bhūmau śayanaṃ vidadhyān mṛdvāstaraṇopapannam | tadadhyāsīta sā||

tāṃ tataḥ samantataḥ parivārya yathoktaguṇāḥ striyaḥ paryupāsīrann āśvāsayantyo vāgbhir grāhiṇīyābhiḥ sāntvanīyābhiś ca ||37||

Suśrutasaṃhitā Śārīrasthāna 10.8

aśankanīyāś catasraḥ striyaḥ pariṇatavayasaḥ prajananakuśalāḥ kartitanakhāḥ paricareyur iti ||8||

Wet-nurses

Kāśyapasaṃhitā Cikitsasthāna 18.63

dhātrī putraśarīrārthaṃ svaśarīropaśoṣaṇam |
snehāt prāpnoti subahūn kleśāṃś cānyān sudāruṇān ||63||

Suśrutasaṃhitā Śārīrasthāna 10.25 (first part)

tato yathāvarṇaṃ dhātrīm upeyān madhyamapramāṇāṃ madhyamavayaskām arogāṃ śīlavatīm acapalām alolupām akṛśām asthūlāṃ prasannakṣīrām alambauṣṭhīm alambordhvastanīm avyaṅgām avyasaninīṃ jīvadvatsāṃ dogdhrīṃ vatsalām akṣudrakarmiṇīṃ kule jātām ato bhūyiṣṭhaiś ca guṇair anvitāṃ śyāmām ārogyabalavṛddhaye bālasya |

Those Who Know Plants

Carakasaṃhitā Sūtrasthāna 1.120–123

oṣadhir nāmarūpābhyāṃ jānate hy ajapā vane |
avipāś caiva gopāś ca ye cānye vanavāsinaḥ ||120||
na nāmajñānamātreṇa rūpajñānena vā punaḥ |
oṣadhīnāṃ parāṃ prāptiṃ kaścid veditum arhati ||121||
yogavit tv apy arūpajñas tāsāṃ tattvavid ucyate |
kiṃ punar yo vijānīyād oṣadhīḥ sarvathā bhiṣak ||122||
yogam āsāṃ tu yo vidyād deśakālopapāditam |
puruṣaṃ puruṣaṃ vīkṣya sa jñeyo bhiṣaguttamaḥ ||123||

Suśrutasaṃhitā Sūtrasthāna 36.10

gopālās tāpasā vyādhā ye cānye vanacāriṇaḥ |
mūlāhārāś ca ye tebhyo bheṣajavyaktir iṣyate ||10||

APPENDIX B

On Becoming a Physician

The Preliminaries of Medical Education

Identifying the Best Materials for Studying

Carakasaṃhitā Vimānasthāna 8.3

buddhimān ātmanaḥ kāryagurulāghavaṃ karmaphalam anubandhaṃ deśakālau ca viditvā yuktidarśanād bhiṣagbubhūṣuḥ śāstram evāditaḥ parīkṣeta | vividhāni hi śāstrāṇi bhiṣajāṃ pracaranti loke; tatra yan manyeta sumahadyaśasvi dhīrapuruṣāsevitam arthabahulam āptajanapūjitaṃ trividhaśiṣyabuddhihitam apagatapunaruktadoṣam ārṣaṃ supraṇītasūtrabhāṣyasaṃgrahakramaṃ svādhāram anavapatitaśabdam akaṣṭaśabdaṃ puṣkalābhidhānaṃ kramāgatārtham arthatattvaviniścayapradhānaṃ saṃgatārtham asaṃkulaprakaraṇam āśuprabodhakaṃ lakṣaṇavac codāharaṇavac ca, tad abhiprapadyeta śāstram | śāstraṃ hy evaṃvidham amala ivādityas tamo vidhūya prakāśayati sarvam ||3||

Choosing the Teacher

Carakasaṃhitā Vimānasthāna 8.4–6

tato 'nantaram ācāryaṃ parīkṣeta; tadyathā– paryavadātaśrutaṃ paridṛṣṭakarmāṇaṃ dakṣaṃ dakṣiṇaṃ śuciṃ jitahastam upakaraṇavantaṃ sarvendriyopapannaṃ prakṛtijñaṃ pratipattijñam[504] anupaskṛtavidyam anahaṅkṛtam anasūyakam akopanaṃ kleśakṣamaṃ śiṣyavatsalam adhyāpakaṃ jñāpanasamarthaṃ ceti | evaṃguṇo hy ācāryaḥ sukṣetram ārtavo megha iva śasyaguṇaiḥ suśiṣyam āśu vaidyaguṇaiḥ saṃpādayati ||4||

tam upasṛtyārirādhayiṣur upacared agnivac ca devavac ca rājavac ca pitṛvac ca bhartṛvac cāpramattaḥ | tatas tatprasādāt kṛtsnaṃ śāstram adhigamya śāstrasya dṛḍhatāyām abhidhānasya sauṣṭhave 'rthasya vijñāne vacanaśaktau ca bhūyo bhūyaḥ prayateta samyak ||5||

tatropāyān anuvyākhyāsyāmaḥ—

adhyayanam adhyāpanaṃ tadvidyasaṃbhāṣā cety upāyāḥ ||6||

Kāśyapasaṃhitā Vimānasthāna 2(?).5

atha guruḥ—dharmajñānavijñānohāpohapratipattikuśalo guṇasampannaḥ saumyadarśanaḥ śuciḥ śiṣyahitadarśī copadeṣṭā ca bhiṣakśāstravyākhyānakuśalas tīrthāgata jñānavijñānaḥ kalyo 'nanyakarmāvyāvṛttaḥ śiṣyaguṇānvitaś ca | ato 'nyathā dauṣer varjyaḥ ||5||

Undertaking Studies

Carakasaṃhitā Vimānasthāna 8.7

tatrāyam adhyayanavidhiḥ—

kalyaḥ kṛtakṣaṇaḥ prātar utthāyopavyūṣaṃ vā kṛtvāvaśyakam upaspṛśyodakaṃ devarṣigobrāhmaṇaguruvṛddhasiddhācāryebhyo namaskṛtya same śucau deśe sukhopaviṣṭo manaḥpuraḥsarābhir vāgbhiḥ sūtram anukrāman punaḥ punar āvartayed buddhvā samyag anupraviśyārthatattvaṃ svadoṣaparihārārthaṃ paradoṣa-pramāṇārthaṃ ca evaṃ madhyaṃdine 'parāhṇe rātrau ca śaśvadaparihāpayann adhyayanam abhyasyet | ity adhyayanavidhiḥ ||7||

Suśrutasaṃhitā Sūtrasthāna 3.54–55

atha vatsa, tad etad adhyeyaṃ yathā tathopadhāraya mayā procyamānaṃ—atha śucaye kṛtottarāsaṅgāyāvyākulāyopasthitāyādhyanakāle śiṣyāya yathāśakti gurur upadiśet padaṃ pādaṃ ślokaṃ vā, te ca padapādaślokā bhūyaḥ krameṇānusaṃdheyāḥ, evam ekaikaśo ghaṭayed ātmanā cānupaṭhet adrutam avilambitam aviśaṅkitam ananunāsikaṃ suvyaktākṣaram apīḍitavarṇam akṣibhruvauṣṭha-hastair anabhinītaṃ susaṃskṛtaṃ nātyuccair nātinīcaiś ca svaraiḥ paṭhet na cāntareṇa kaścid vrajet tayor adhīyānayoḥ ||54|| bhavataś cātra—

śucir guruparo dakṣas tandrānidrāvivarjitaḥ paṭhann etena vidhinā, śiṣyaḥ śāstrāntam āpnuyāt ||55||

Suśrutasaṃhitā Sūtrasthāna 4.3–4

adhigatam apy adhyayanam aprabhāṣitam arthataḥ kharasya candanabhāra iva kevalaṃ pariśramakaraṃ bhavati ||3||

bhavati cātra—

yathā kharaś candanabhāravāhī bhārasya vettā na tu candanasya |
evaṃ hi śāstrāṇi bahūny adhītya cārtheṣu mūḍhāḥ kharavad vahanti ||4||

Choosing the Student

Carakasaṃhitā Vimānasthāna 8.8

athādhyāpanavidhiḥ—

adhyāpane kṛtabuddhir ācāryaḥ śiṣyam evāditaḥ parīkṣeta tadyathā praśāntam āryaprakṛtikam akṣudrakarmāṇam ṛjucakṣurmukhanāsā-vaṃśaṃ tanu-raktaviśadajihvam avikṛtadantauṣṭham aminminaṃ dhṛtimantam anahaṅkṛtaṃ medhāvinaṃ vitarkasmṛtisaṃpannam udārasattvaṃ tadvidyakulajam athavā tadvidyavṛttaṃ tattvābhiniveśinam avyaṅgam avyāpannendriyaṃ nibhṛtam anuddhatam arthatattvabhāvakam akopanam avyasaninaṃ śīlaśaucā-cārānurāgadākṣyaprādakṣiṇyopapannam adhyayanābhikāmam arthavijñāne karmadarśane cānanyakāryam alubdham analasaṃ sarvabhūtahitaiṣiṇam ācārya-sarvānuśiṣṭipratikaram anuraktaṃ ca evaṃguṇasamuditam adhyāpyam āhuḥ ||8||

Suśrutasaṃhitā Sūtrasthāna 2.1–3

athātaḥ śiṣyopanayanīyam adhyāyaṃ vyākhyāsyāmaḥ ||1||
yathovāca bhagavān dhanvantariḥ ||2||
brāhmaṇakṣatriyavaiśyānām anyatamam anvayavayaḥśīlaśauryaśaucācāravinaya-śaktibala medhādhṛtismṛtimatipratipattiyuktaṃ tanujihvauṣṭhadantāgram ṛju-vaktrākṣināsaṃ prasannacittavākceṣṭaṃ kleśasahaṃ ca bhiṣak śiṣyam upanayet ato viparīta guṇaṃ nopanayet ||3||

Aṣṭāṅgasaṃgraha Sūtrasthāna 2.2–4ab

gurubhakto 'bhiyukto 'tiyukto dhīsmṛtipāṭavaiḥ |
ṛjvāsyanāsānayanas tanusnigdhanakhacchaviḥ ||2||
brahmacārī jitadvandvo dhīraḥ sucaritaḥ sthiraḥ |
ṣaṇmāsān uṣitaḥ śukle lajjāśaucakulānvitaḥ ||3||
śiṣyo 'dhyāpyo gato yāvadantaṃ tantrārthakarmaṇām |

Kāśyapasaṃhitā Vimānasthāna 2(?).4

atha śiṣyagunāḥ—
kṣāntir dākṣyaṃ dākṣiṇyam ānukūlyaṃ śaucaṃ kule janma dharmasatyāhiṃsā-sāmakalyāṇajñānavijñānasthitiviniveśaḥ pāṭavaṃ yathoktakāritvaṃ brahmacaryam anutseko lobherṣyāvivarjanam iti; ato 'nyathā doṣaiḥ sa varjyaḥ ||4||

The Initiation of the Medical Student

Carakasaṃhitā Vimānasthāna 8.9–14

evaṃvidham adhyayanārthinam upasthitam ārirādhayiṣum ācāryo 'nubhāṣeta udagayane śuklapakṣe praśaste 'hani tiṣyahastaśravaṇāśvayujām anyatamena nakṣatreṇa yogam upagate bhagavati śaśini kalyāṇe kalyāṇe ca karaṇe maitre muhūrte[505] muṇḍaḥ kṛtopavāsaḥ snātaḥ kāṣāyavastrasaṃvītaḥ sagandhahastaḥ samidho 'gnim ājyam upalepanam udakumbhān mālyadāmadīpahiraṇyahemarajatamaṇi-muktāvidrumakṣaumaparidhīn kuśalājasarṣapākṣatāṃś ca śuklāni sumanāṃsi grathitāgrathitāni medhyān bhakṣyān gandhāṃś ca ghṛṣṭān ādāyopatiṣṭhasveti ||9||
sa tathā kuryāt ||10||
tam upasthitam ājñāya same śucau deśe prākpravaṇe udakpravaṇe vā catuṣ-kiṣkumātraṃ caturasraṃ sthaṇḍilaṃ gomayodakenopaliptaṃ kuśāstīrṇaṃ suparihitaṃ paridhibhiś caturdiśaṃ yathoktacandanodakumbhakṣaumahema-hiraṇyarajatamaṇimuktāvidrumālaṅkṛtaṃ medhyabhakṣyagandhaśuklapuṣpa-lājasarṣapākṣatopaśobhitaṃ kṛtvā, tatra pālāśībhir aiṅgudībhir audumbarībhir mādhūkībhir vā samidbhir agnim upasamādhāya prāṅmukhaḥ śucir adhyayana-vidhim anuvidhāya madhusarpirbhyāṃ tris trir juhuyād agnim *āśīḥ* saṃprayuktair

mantrair brahmāṇam agniṃ dhanvantariṃ prajāpatim aśvināv indram ṛṣīṃś ca sūtrakārān abhimantrayamāṇaḥ pūrvaṃ svāheti ||11||
śiṣyaś cainam anvālabheta hutvā ca pradakṣiṇam agnim anuparikrāmet parikramya brāhmaṇān svasti vācayet bhiṣajaś cābhipūjayet ||12||
athainam agnisakāśe brāhmaṇasakāśe bhiṣaksakāśe cānuśiṣyāt—
brahmacāriṇā śmaśrudhāriṇā satyavādināmāṃsādena medhyasevinā nirmatsareṇāśastradhāriṇā ca bhavitavyaṃ,[506] na ca te madvacanāt kiñcid akāryaṃ syād anyatra rājadviṣṭāt prāṇaharād vipulād adharmyād anarthasaṃprayuktād vāpy arthāt; madarpaṇena matpradhānena madadhīnena matpriyahitānuvartinā ca śaśvad bhavitavyaṃ, putravad dāsavad arthivac copacaratānuvastavyo 'ham, anutsekenāvahitenānanyamanasā vinītenāvekṣyāvekṣyakāriṇānasūyakena cābhyanujñātena pravicaritavyam, anujñātena pravicaratā pūrvaṃ gurvarthopāharaṇe yathāśakti prayatitavyaṃ, karmasiddhim arthasiddhiṃ yaśolābhaṃ pretya ca svargam icchatā bhiṣajā tvayā gobrāhmaṇam ādau kṛtvā sarvaprāṇabhṛtāṃ śarmāśāsitavyam aharahar uttiṣṭhatā copaviśatā ca, sarvātmanā cāturāṇām ārogyāya prayatitavyaṃ, jīvitahetor api cāturebhyo nābhidrogdhavyaṃ, manasāpi ca parastriyo nābhigamanīyās tathā sarvam eva parasvaṃ, nibhṛtaveśaparicchadena bhavitavyam, aśauṇḍenāpāpenāpāpasahāyena ca, ślakṣṇaśukladharmyaśarmyadhanyasatyahitamitavacasā deśakālavicāriṇā smṛtimatā jñānotthānopakaraṇasaṃpatsu nityaṃ yatnavatā ca;
na ca kadācid rājadviṣṭānāṃ rājadveṣiṇāṃ vā mahājanadviṣṭānāṃ mahājanadveṣiṇāṃ vāpy auṣadham anuvidhātavyaṃ, tathā sarveṣām atyarthavikṛtaduṣṭaduḥkhaśīlācāropacārāṇām anapavādapratikārāṇāṃ mumūrṣūṇāṃ ca, tathaivāsannihiteśvarāṇāṃ strīṇām anadhyakṣāṇāṃ vā;
na ca kadācit strīdattam āmiṣam ādātavyam ananujñātaṃ bhartrāthavādhyakṣeṇa, āturakulaṃ cānupraviśatā viditenānumatapraveśinā sārdhaṃ puruṣeṇa susaṃvītenāvākśirasā smṛtimatā stimitenāvekṣyāvekṣya manasā sarvam ācaratā samyag anupraveṣṭavyam, anupraviśya ca vāṅmanobuddhīndriyāṇi na kvacit praṇidhātavyāny anyatrāturād āturopakārārthād āturagateṣv anyeṣu vā bhāveṣu, na cāturakulapravṛttayo bahir niścārayitavyāḥ, hrasitaṃ cāyuṣaḥ pramāṇam āturasya jānatāpi tvayā na varṇayitavyaṃ tatra yatrocyamānam āturasyānyasya vāpy upaghātāya saṃpadyate;
jñānavatāpi ca nātyartham ātmano jñāne vikatthitavyam āptād api hi vikatthamānād atyartham udvijanty aneke ||13||
na caiva hy asti sutaram āyurvedasya pāraṃ, tasmād apramattaḥ śaśvad abhiyogam asmin gachet, etac ca kāryam, evaṃbhūyaś ca vṛttasauṣṭhavam anasūyatā parebhyo 'py āgamayitavyaṃ, kṛtsno hi loko buddhimatām ācāryaḥ śatruś cābuddhimatām, ataś cābhisamīkṣya buddhimatāmitrasyāpi dhanyaṃ yaśasyam āyuṣyaṃ pauṣṭikaṃ laukyam abhyupadiśato vacaḥ śrotavyam anuvidhātavyaṃ ceti | ataḥ param idaṃ brūyāt—
devatāgnidvijaguruvṛddhasiddhācāryeṣu te nityaṃ samyag vartitavyaṃ, teṣu te samyag vartamānasyāyam agniḥ sarvagandharasaratnabījāni yatheritāś ca devatāḥ

śivāya syuḥ, ato 'nyathā vartamānasyāśivāyeti | evaṃ bruvati cācārye śiṣyaḥ tatheti brūyāt | yathopadeśaṃ ca kurvann adhyāpyaḥ, ato 'nyathā tv anadhyāpyaḥ | adhyāpyam adhyāpayan hy ācāryo yathoktaiś cādhyāpanaphalair yogam āpnoty anyaiś cānuktaiḥ śreyaskarair guṇaiḥ śiṣyam ātmānaṃ ca yunakti | ity adhyāpanavidhir uktaḥ ||14||

Suśrutasaṃhitā Sūtrasthāna 2.4–10

upanayanīyaṃ tu brāhmaṇaṃ praśasteṣu tithikaraṇamuhūrtanakṣatreṣu praśastāyāṃ diśi śucau same deśe caturhastaṃ caturasraṃ sthaṇḍilam upalipya gomayena, darbhaiḥ saṃstīrya, ratnapuṣpalājabhaktair devatāḥ pūjayitvā viprān bhiṣajaś ca, tatrollikhyābhyukṣya ca dakṣiṇato brahmāṇaṃ sthāpayitvāgnim upasamādhāya, khadirapalāśadevadārubilvānāṃ samidbhiś caturṇāṃ vā kṣīrivṛkṣāṇāṃ (nyagrodhodumbarāśvatthamadhūkānāṃ) dadhimadhughṛtāktābhir dārvīhaumikena vidhinā sapraṇavābhir mahāvyāhṛtibhiḥ sruveṇājyāhutīr juhuyāt, tataḥ pratidaivatam ṛṣīṃś ca svāhākāraṃ kuryāt, śiṣyam api kārayet ||4||

brāhmaṇas trayāṇāṃ varṇānām upanayanaṃ kartum arhati, (rājanyo dvayasya, vaiśyo vaiśyasyaiveti), śūdram api kulaguṇasampannaṃ mantravarjam anupanītam adhyāpayed ity eke ||5||

tato 'gniṃ triḥ pariṇīyāgnisākṣikaṃ śiṣyaṃ brūyāt kāmakrodhalobhamohamānāhaṅkārerṣyāpāruṣya paiśunyānṛtālasyāyaśasyāni hitvā, nīcanakharomṇā śucinā kaṣāyavāsasā satyavratabrahmacaryābhivādanatatpareṇāvaśyaṃ bhavitavyaṃ, madanumatasthānagamanaśayanāsanabhojanādhyayanapareṇa bhūtvā matpriyahiteṣu vartitavyam, ato 'nyathā te vartamānasyādharmo bhavati, aphalā ca vidyā, na ca prākāśyaṃ prāpnoti ||6||

ahaṃ vā tvayi samyag vartamāne yady anyathādarśī syām enobhāg bhaveyam aphalavidyaś ca ||7||

dvijagurudaridramitrapravrajitopanatasādhvanāthābhyupagatānāṃ cātmabāndhavānām iva svabhaiṣajaiḥ pratikartavyam, evaṃ sādhu bhavati, vyādhaśākunikapatitapāpakāriṇāṃ ca na pratikartavyam, evaṃ vidyā prakāśate mitrayaśodharmārthakāmāṃś ca prāpnoti ||8||

bhavataś cātra—

kṛṣṇe 'ṣṭamī tannidhane 'hanī dve śukle tathāpy evam ahardvisandhyam akālavidyutstanayitnughoṣe svatantrarāṣṭrakṣitipavyathāsu ||9||

śmaśānayānādyatanāhaveṣu mahotsavautpātikadarśaneṣu nādhyeyam anyeṣu ca yeṣu viprā nādhīyate nāśucinā ca nityam ||10||

Kāśyapasaṃhitā Vimānasthāna 2(?).3

atha khalu guruḥ śiṣyam abhigataṃ vidyārthinaṃ śiṣyaguṇānvitaṃ vidhinopanayed udagayane puṇyāhe nakṣatre 'śvayuji rohiṇyām uttarāsv anyasmin vā | puṇye prāgudakpravaṇadeśe gomayenādbhiś ca gocarmamātraṃ sthaṇḍilam upalipya; yathoktaṃ tatra lakṣaṇollekhanāgnipraṇayanaparisamūhanaparyukṣaṇabrahmapraṇītāstaraṇājyotpavanāghārājyabhāgāgnihomān kṛtvā, pālāśīḥ samidho ghṛtāktā juhoti—agnaye svāhā, somāya svāhā, prajāpataye svāhā, kaśyapāya svāhā, aśvibhyāṃ svāhā, indrāya svāhā, dhanvantaraye svāhā, sarasvatyai svāhā, pūrṇabhagāya svāhā, agnaye sviṣṭakṛte svāhā, iti hutvā; brāhmaṇaṃ huviṣyaudanena dakṣiṇāvatā tarpayitvā, devāṃś ca balibhiḥ, gurave pūrṇakumbhaṃ dakṣiṇāṃ dattvā, 'dadhikrāvṇa' iti prāṅmukho dadhi prāśya, upaspṛśyādbhiḥ, parikramya pradakṣiṇam, guror bāhuṃ saṃspṛśya brūyāt—asāv ahaṃ putra iti, pādau saṃspṛśya brūyāt—asāv ahaṃ śiṣya iti ||3||

Kāśyapasaṃhitā Vimānasthāna 2(?).6

atha śiṣyānuśāsanaṃ– bhoḥ saumyenānukūlena dharmikeṇa jitendriyeṇāhūtādhyāyinā ca bhavitavyaṃ, sarvanivedinā samānaduḥkhena deśakālajñena dhṛtimatā ca bhavitavyaṃ, lobhakrodhamoherṣyāprahāsavairamadyamāṃsastrībhyo nivarttitavyaṃ, guruśuśrūṣāvaśeṣeṇādhyetavyaṃ, na cānanujñātena na cānabhyarcya vā gurum asamāptavidyena vā pracāritavyam ||6||

Aṣṭāṅgasaṃgraha Sūtrasthāna 2.6–7a

hīnānyaveṣa ācāryaṃ paryupāsīta rājavat | śayīta supta evāsminn uttiṣṭhetāsya pūrvataḥ ||6||
na brūyāt kevalaṃ nāma nāsādhv api vināṭayet |

The Suśrutasaṃhitā on Physicians' Professional Conduct

Suśrutasaṃhitā Sūtrasthāna 10.3–4, 6, and 8

adhigatatantreṇopāsitatantrārthena dṛṣṭakarmaṇā kṛtayogyena śāstraṃ nigadatā rājānujñātena nīcanakharomṇā śucinā śuklavastraparihitena chatravatā daṇḍahastena sopānatkenānuddhataveśena sumanasā kalyāṇābhivyāhāreṇākuhakena bandhubhūtena bhūtānāṃ susahāyavatā vaidyena viśikhānupraveṣṭavyā ||3||
tato dūtanimittaśakunamaṅgalānulomyenāturagṛham abhigamya, upaviśya, āturam abhipaśyet spṛśet pṛcchec ca, tribhir etair vijñānopāyai rogāḥ prāyaśo veditavyā ity eke, tat tu na samyak, ṣaḍvidho hi rogāṇāṃ vijñānopāyaḥ, tadyathā pañcabhiḥ śrotrādibhiḥ praśnena ceti ||4||
(...)
evam abhisamīkṣya sādhyān sādhayet, yāpyān yāpayet, asādhyān naivopakrameta, parisaṃvatsarotthitāṃś ca vikārān prāyaśo varjayet ||6||
(...)
tatra sādhyā api vyādhayaḥ prāyeṇaiṣāṃ duścikitsyatamā bhavanti tadyathā śrotriyanṛpatistrībālavṛddhabhīrurājasevakakitavadurbalavaidyavidagdhavyādhigopakadaridrakṛpaṇakrodhanānām anātmavatām anāthānāṃ ca, evaṃ nirūpya cikitsāṃ kurvan dharmārthakāmayaśāṃsi prāpnoti ||8||
bhavati cātra—
strībhiḥ sahāsyāṃ saṃvāsaṃ parihāsaṃ ca varjayet ||
dattaṃ ca tābhyo nādeyam annād anyad bhiṣagvaraiḥ ||9||

The Kāśyapasaṃhitā on Physicians' Professional Conduct

Kāśyapasaṃhitā Vimānasthāna 2.(?)8

adhītyānujñātaḥ pracarec chuklavāsāḥ saṃhatakeśo[507] 'nudbhrānto yugamātrāvalokī pūrvābhibhāṣī sumukhaḥ | na cāturakulam anāhūtaḥ praviśet, praviśaṃś ca nimittāni lakṣayet | na ca sarvato 'valokayed anyatrāturāt | na cāturakuleṣu strībhiḥ preṣyābhir api sahopahāsaṃ gacchet, na cāsām apūjāpuraskṛtaṃ nāma gṛhṇīyāt, mānyasthānenaiva tu brūyāt, na ca tābhiḥ saṃvyavahāram atipraṇayaṃ vā kuryāt, na ca bhartur aviditaṃ strībhyaḥ kiñcid ādadyāt, na cāviditaḥ praviśet,[508] na ca rahasi striyā saha brūyād āsīta vā, na caināṃ vivṛtāṃ prekṣeta vihased vā, praṇayantīṃ copekṣeta, na ca prakāśayet | na cāturakulaguhyaṃ bahiḥ prakāśayet, nāturakuladoṣān prathayet | dṛṣṭāriṣṭam api cāturaṃ na tattvaṃ brūyāt, nityam āśvāsayet | na mṛtyuparigataśarīram asādhyarogam anupakaraṇaṃ copagacchet, nauṣadham akrameṇopadiśet, na parādhīnaṃ kuryāt | na svayaṃ kṛtakam auṣadhaṃ prayuñjīta, śarīrauṣadhavyādhivayasāṃ cāvasthāntarajñaḥ syāt | nityasaṃbhṛtadhūpāñjanauṣadhaḥ syāt | na cānyabhiṣagbhir virodhaṃ gacchet | saṃyuktaś ca tair auṣadhaṃ prakalpayet | pragalbho niḥśaṅka upasthitapade vispaṣṭaṃ vicitraṃ mṛdūpanayavad grāhakam aviruddhaṃ dharmyaṃ sadā brūyāt | prajānāṃ hi svastikāmo bhiṣag iha cāmutra ca nandata iti ||8||

The Aṣṭāṅgasaṃgraha on Physicians' Professional Conduct

Aṣṭāṅgasaṃgraha Sūtrasthāna 2.7cd–20

abhedyo 'nuddhataḥ stabdhaḥ sūnṛtaḥ priyadarśanaḥ ||7cd||
bahuśrutaḥ kālavedī jñātagrantho 'rthaśāstravit |
anāthān rogiṇo yaś ca putravat samupācaret ||8||
guruṇā samanujñātaḥ sa bhiṣakśabdam aśnute |
yas tu kevalaśāstrajñaḥ karmasvapariniṣṭhitaḥ ||9||
sa muhyaty āturaṃ prāpya prāpya bhīrur ivāhavam |
yaḥ punaḥ kurute karma dhārṣṭyāc chāstravivarjitaḥ ||10||
sa satsu garhām āpnoti vadhaṃ carcchati rājataḥ |
hetau liṅge praśamane rogāṇām apunarbhave ||11||
jñānaṃ caturvidhaṃ yasya sa rājārho bhiṣaktamaḥ |
śastraṃ śāstrāṇi salilaṃ guṇadoṣapravṛttaye ||12||
pātrāpekṣiṇy ataḥ prajñāṃ bāhuśrutyena bṛṃhayet |
pradīpabhūtaṃ śāstraṃ hi darśanaṃ vipulā matiḥ ||13||
tābhyāṃ bhiṣak suyuktābhyāṃ cikitsan nāparādhyati |
āhūta eva yo yāti suveṣaḥ sunimittaḥ ||14||
gatvāturārthād anyatra na nidhatte manaḥ kacit |
vyādhīn parīkṣate samyaṅ nidānādiviśeṣataḥ ||15||
hreṣaṇīyāṃ ca tadvārttāṃ na prakāśayate bahiḥ |

sahasā na ca tasyāpi kriyākālam ahāpayan ||16||
jānāti copacaritum sa vaidyaḥ siddhim aśnute |
nādadītāmiṣaṃ strībhyas tadadhyakṣe parāṅmukhe ||17||
tābhiś ca rahasi sthānaṃ parihāsaṃ ca varjayet |
ārtaṃ ca nṛpasadvaidyair dviṣṭaṃ tadveṣiṇaṃ dviṣam ||18||
caṇḍaṃ śokāturaṃ bhīruṃ kṛtaghnaṃ vaidyamāninam|
hīnopakaraṇaṃ vyagram avidheyaṃ gatāyuṣam ||19||
jijīviṣur vyādhito 'pi pūrvoktaguṇavarjitān |
kriyāvikrayiṇo vaidyān mṛtyor agresarā hi te ||20||

APPENDIX C

On Continued Learning and Interaction with Peers

Suśrutasaṃhitā Sūtrasthāna 3.56

vāksauṣṭhave 'rthavijñāne prāgalbhye karmanaipuṇe ||
tadabhyāse ca siddhau ca yatetādhyayanāntagaḥ ||56||

Carakasaṃhitā Vimānasthāna 8.15

saṃbhāṣāvidhim ata ūrdhvaṃ vyākhyāsyāmaḥ—bhiṣak bhiṣajā saha saṃbhāṣeta | tadvidyasaṃbhāṣā hi jñānābhiyogasaṃharṣakarī bhavati, vaiśāradyam api cābhinirvartayati, vacanaśaktim api cādhatte, yaśaś cābhidīpayati, pūrvaśrute ca saṃdehavataḥ punaḥ śravaṇāc chrutasaṃśayam apakarṣati, śrute cāsaṃdehavato bhūyo 'dhyavasāyam abhinirvartayati, aśrutam api ca kañcid arthaṃ śrotraviṣayam āpādayati, yac cācāryaḥ śiṣyāya śuśrūṣave prasannaḥ krameṇopadiśati guhyābhimatam arthajātaṃ tat parasparеṇa saha jalpan piṇḍena vijigīṣur āha saṃharṣāt, tasmāt tadvidyasaṃbhāṣām abhipraśaṃsanti kuśalāḥ ||15||

Carakasaṃhitā Vimānasthāna 8.67

vādas tu khalu bhiṣajāṃ pravartamāno pravartet āyurveda eva, nānyatra | atra hi vākyaprativākyavistarāḥ kevalāś copapattayaḥ sarvādhikaraṇeṣu | tāḥ sarvāḥ samavekṣyāvekṣya sarvaṃ vākyaṃ brūyāt, nāprakṛtakam aśāstram aparīkṣitam asādhakam ākulam avyāpakaṃ vā | sarvaṃ ca hetumad brūyāt | hetumanto hy akaluṣāḥ sarva eva vādavigrahāś cikitsite kāraṇabhūtāḥ, praśastabuddhivardhakatvāt; sarvārambhasiddhiṃ hy āvahaty anupahatā buddhiḥ ||67||

APPENDIX D

To Care or Not to Care

The Signs of Impending Death

Aṣṭāṅgahṛdayasaṃhitā Śārīrasthāna 5.131

āyurvedaphalaṃ kṛtsnaṃ yad āyurjñe pratiṣṭhitam |
riṣṭajñānādṛtas tasmāt sarvadaiva bhaved bhiṣak ||131||

Disease Classification

Aṣṭāṅgasaṃgraha Śārīrasthāna 7.30–31ab

puṇyavān niyatāyuś cana kathañcin na jīvati | tasmād ācaram occhvāsāc cikitsed eva yatnataḥ ||30|| tadbandhumitrānumataḥ pratyākhyāyāturaṃ bhiṣak ||31||

On the Reasons Not to Treat Terminally Ill Patients

Carakasaṃhitā Indriyasthāna 11.27

pādāḥ sametāś catvāraḥ, saṃpannāḥ sādhakair guṇaiḥ |
vyarthā gatāyuṣo dravyaṃ, vinā nāsti guṇodayaḥ ||27||

Aṣṭāṅgahṛdayasaṃhitā Śārīrasthāna 5.130

yamadūtapiśācādyair yat parāsur upāsyate |
ghnadbhir auṣadhavīryāṇi tasmāt taṃ parivarjayet ||130||

Carakasaṃhitā Sūtrasthāna 10.7–8

sādhyāsādhyavibhāgajño jñānapūrvaṃ cikitsakaḥ |
kāle cārabhate karma yat tat sādhayati dhruvam ||7||
arthavidyāyaśohānim upakrośam asaṃgraham |
prāpnuyān niyataṃ vaidyo yo 'sādhyaṃ samupācaret ||8||

Suśrutasaṃhitā Sūtrasthāna 28.7

asiddhim āpnuyāl loke pratikurvan gatāyuṣaḥ ||
ato 'riṣṭāni yatnena lakṣayet kuśalo bhiṣak ||7||

A License to Care

Carakasaṃhitā Cikitsāsthāna 13.175–178

kriyātivṛtte jaṭhare tridoṣe cāpraśāmyati ||175||
jñātīn sasuhṛdo dārān brāhmaṇān nṛpatīn gurūn|
anujñāpya bhiṣak karma vidadhyāt saṃśayaṃ bravan ||176||
akriyāyāṃ dhruvo mṛtyuḥ kriyāyāṃ saṃśayo bhavet|
evam ākhyāya tasyedam anujñātaḥ suhṛdgaṇaiḥ ||177||
pānabhojanasaṃyuktaṃ viṣam asmai prayojayet|
yasmin vā kupitaḥ sarpo visṛjed dhi phale viṣam ||178||

APPENDIX E

The Rewards of Medical Practice

Carakasaṃhitā Sūtrasthāna 15.19–21

daridras tv āpadaṃ prāpya prāptakālaṃ viśodhanam | pibet kāmam asaṃbhṛtya saṃbhārān api durlabhān ||19||
na hi sarvamanuṣyāṇāṃ santi sarve paricchadāḥ | na ca rogā na bādhante daridrān api dāruṇāḥ ||20||
yad yac chakyaṃ manuṣyeṇa kartum auṣadham āpadi | tat tat sevyaṃ yathāśakti vasanāny aśanāni ca ||21||

Aṣṭāṅgasaṃgraha Uttarasthāna 50.192

na jīvitapradānād dhi dānam anyad viśiṣyate | tasmād upācaret svena svena niḥsvatapasvinaḥ ||192||

Carakasaṃhitā Sūtrasthāna 30.29

sa cādhyetavyo brāhmaṇarājanyavaiśyaiḥ | tatrānugrahārthaṃ prāṇināṃ brāhmaṇaiḥ, ārakṣārthaṃ rājanyaiḥ, vṛttyarthaṃ vaiśyaiḥ, sāmānyato vā dharmārthakāmaparigrahārthaṃ sarvaiḥ | tatra yad adhyātmavidāṃ dharmapathasthānāṃ dharmaprakāśakānāṃ vā mātṛpitṛbhrātṛbandhugurujanasya vā vikārapraśamane prayatnavān bhavati, yac cāyurvedoktam adhyātmam anudhyāyati vedayaty anuvidhīyate vā so 'sya paro dharmaḥ, yā punar īśvarāṇāṃ vasumatāṃ vā sakāśāt sukhopahāranimittā bhavaty arthāvāptir ārakṣaṇaṃ ca, yā ca svaparigṛhītānāṃ prāṇinām āturyād ārakṣā, so 'syārthaḥ; yat punar asya vidvadgrahaṇayaśaḥ śaraṇyatvaṃ ca, yā ca saṃmānaśuśrūṣā, yac ceṣṭānāṃ viṣayāṇām ārogyam ādhatte so 'sya kāmaḥ | iti yathāpraśnam uktam aśeṣeṇa ||29||

Kāśyapasaṃhitā Vimānasthāna 2.10 (middle part)

kena cādhyeya iti, brāhmaṇakṣatriyavaiśyaśūdrair āyurvedo adhyeyaḥ || tatrārthaṃ parijñānārthaṃ puṇyārthaṃ cātmanaḥ prajānugrahārthaṃ brāhmaṇaiḥ, prajāsaṃrakṣaṇārthaṃ kṣatriyaiḥ, vṛttyarthaṃ vaiśyaiḥ, śuśrūṣārtham itaraiḥ dharmārthaṃ ca sarvaiḥ |

Bhāvaprakāśa Pūrvakhaṇḍa 6.34–35

naiva kurvīta lobhena cikitsāpuṇyavikrayam |
īśvarāṇāṃ vasumatāṃ lipsetārthaṃ tu vṛttaye ||34||

cikitsitaṃ śarīraṃ yo na niṣkrīṇāti durmatiḥ |
sa yat karoti sukṛtaṃ sarvaṃ tad bhiṣag aśnute ||35||

Carakasaṃhitā Sūtrasthāna 5.104

vṛttyupāyān niṣeveta ye syur dharmāvirodhinaḥ | śamam adhyayanaṃ caiva sukham evaṃ samaśnute ||104||

Carakasaṃhitā Sūtrasthāna 11.5

atha dvitīyāṃ dhanaiṣaṇām āpadyeta, prāṇebhyo hy anantaraṃ dhanam eva paryeṣṭavyaṃ bhavati; na hy ataḥ pāpāt pāpīyo 'sti yad anupakaraṇasya dīrgham āyuḥ, tasmād upakaraṇāni paryeṣṭuṃ yateta | tatropakaraṇopāyān anuvyākhyāsyāmaḥ tadyathā—kṛṣipāśupālyavāṇijyarājopasevādīni, yāni cānyāny api satām avigarhitāni karmāṇi vṛttipuṣṭikarāṇi vidyāt tāny ārabheta kartuṃ; tathā kurvan dīrghajīvitaṃ jīvaty anavamataḥ puruṣo bhavati | iti dvitīyā dhanaiṣaṇā vyākhyātā bhavati ||5||[509]

Carakasaṃhitā Cikitsāsthāna 1.51–62

śīlavān matimān yukto dvijātiḥ śāstrapāragaḥ |
prāṇibhir guruvat pūjyaḥ prāṇācāryaḥ sa hi smṛtaḥ ||51||
vidyāsamāptau bhiṣajo dvitīyā jātir ucyate |
aśnute vaidyaśabdaṃ hi na vaidyaḥ pūrvajanmanā ||52||
vidyāsamāptau brāhmaṃ vā sattvam ārṣam athāpi vā |
dhruvam āviśati jñānāt tasmād vaidyo dvijaḥ smṛtaḥ ||53||
nābhidhyāyen na cākrośed ahitaṃ na samācaret |
prāṇācāryaṃ budhaḥ kaścid icchann āyuranitvaram ||54||
cikitsitas tu saṃśrutye yo vāsaṃśrutya mānavaḥ |
nopākaroti vaidyāya nāsti tasyeha niṣkṛtiḥ ||55||
bhiṣag apy āturān sarvān svasutān iva yatnavān |
ābādhebhyo hi saṃrakṣed icchan dharmam anuttamam ||56||
dharmārthaṃ cārthakāmārtham āyurvedo maharṣibhiḥ |
prakāśito dharmaparair icchadbhiḥ sthānam akṣaram ||57||
nārthārthaṃ nāpi kāmārtham atha bhūtadayāṃ prati |
vartate yaś cikitsāyāṃ sa sarvam ativartate ||58||
kurvate ye tu vṛttyarthaṃ cikitsāpaṇyavikrayam |
te hitvā kāñcanaṃ rāśiṃ pāṃśurāśim upāsate ||59||
dāruṇaiḥ kṛṣyamāṇānāṃ gadair vaivasvatakṣayam |
chittvā vaivasvatān pāśān jīvitaṃ yaḥ prayacchati ||60||
dharmārthadātā sadṛśas tasya nehopalabhyate |
na hi jīvitadānād dhi dānam anyad viśiṣyate ||61||
paro bhūtadayā dharma iti matvā cikitsayā |
vartate yaḥ sa siddhārthaḥ sukham atyantam aśnute ||62||

Bhāvaprakāśa Pūrvakhaṇḍa 6.32

atha cikitsāyāḥ phalam āha kvacid arthaḥ kvacin maitrī kvacid dharmaḥ kvacid yaśaḥ karmābhyāsaḥ kvacic ceti cikitsā nāsti niṣphalā ||32||

Aṣṭāṅgasaṃgraha Uttarasthāna 50.194

kvaccid dharmaḥ kvacin mitraṃ kvacid arthaḥ kvacid yaśaḥ | karmābhyāsaḥ kvaccic ceti cikitsā nāsti niṣphalā ||194||

APPENDIX F

Veracity in the Doctor–Patient Relationship

The Epistemology of Honesty and Lying in the Ayurvedic Classics

Suśrutasaṃhitā Sūtrasthāna 25.43–44

mātaraṃ pitaraṃ putrān bāndhavān api cāturaḥ ||
apy etān abhiśaṅketa vaidye viśvāsam eti ca ||43||
visṛjaty ātmanātmānaṃ na cainaṃ pariśaṅkate ||
tasmāt putravad evainaṃ pālayed āturaṃ bhiṣak ||44||

Aṣṭāṅgasaṃgraha Uttarasthāna 50.189

bhiṣag apy āturān sarvān svasutān iva yatnavān | ābādhebhyo 'bhisaṃrakṣet jñānaṃ dharmam anusmaran ||189||

Carakasaṃhitā Vimānasthāna 3.24 (latter part)

teṣām udārasattvaguṇakarmaṇām acintyarasavīryavipākaprabhāvaguṇasamuditāni prādurbabhūvuḥ śasyāni sarvaguṇasamuditatvāt pṛthivyādīnāṃ kṛtayugasyādau |
bhraśyati tu kṛtayuge keṣāṃcid atyādānāt sāṃpannikānāṃ sattvānāṃ śarīragauravam āsīt śarīragauravāc chramaḥ śramād ālasyam ālasyāt saṃcayaḥ saṃcayāt parigrahaḥparigrahāl lobhaḥ prādur āsīt kṛte |
tatas tretāyāṃ lobhād abhidrohaḥ abhidrohād anṛtavacanam anṛtavacanāt kāmakrodhamānadveṣapāruṣyābhighātabhayatāpaśokacintodvegādayaḥ pravṛttāḥ |
tatas tretāyāṃ dharmapādo 'ntardhānam agamat |
tasyāntardhānāt yugavarṣapramāṇasya pādahrāsaḥ pṛthivyādeś ca guṇapādapraṇāśo 'bhūt |
tatpraṇāśakṛtaś ca śasyānāṃ snehavaimalyarasavīryavipākaprabhāvaguṇapādabhraṃśaḥ |
tatas tāni prajāśarīrāṇi hīyamānaguṇapādair āhāravihārair ayathāpūrvam upaṣṭabhyamānāny agnimārutaparītāni prāg vyādhibhir jvarādibhir ākrāntāni |
ataḥ prāṇino hrāsam avāpur āyuṣaḥ kramaśa iti ||24||

Suśrutasaṃhitā Śārīrasthāna 1.18

sāttvikās tu—ānṛśaṃsyaṃ saṃvibhāgarucitā titikṣā satyaṃ dharma āstikyaṃ jñānaṃ buddhir medhā smṛtir dhṛtir anabhiṣaṅgaś ca rājasās tu duḥkhabahulatāṭanaśīlatādhṛtir ahaṅkāra ānṛtikatvam akāruṇyaṃ dambho māno harṣaḥ kāmaḥ krodhaś ca tāmasās tu viṣāditvaṃ nāstikyam adharmaśīlatā buddher nirodho 'jñānaṃ durmedhastvam akarmaśīlatā nidrālutvaṃ ceti ||18||

Carakasaṃhitā Sūtrasthāna 1.57–58

vāyuḥ pittaṃ kaphaś coktaḥ śārīro doṣasaṃgrahaḥ |
mānasaḥ punar uddiṣṭo rajaś ca tama eva ca ||57||
praśāmyaty auṣadhaiḥ pūrvo daivayuktivyapāśrayaiḥ |
mānaso jñānavijñānadhairyasmṛtisamādhibhiḥ ||58||

Carakasaṃhitā Cikitsāsthāna 24.72–73

sasyasaṃbodhakaṃ varṣaṃ hemaprakṛtidarśakaḥ |
hutāśaḥ sarvasattvānāṃ madyaṃ tūbhayakārakam ||72||
pradhānāvaramadhyānāṃ rūpāṇāṃ vyaktidarśakaḥ |
yathāgnir evaṃ sattvānāṃ madyaṃ prakṛtidarśakam ||73||

Suśrutasaṃhitā Sūtrasthāna 45.209

aśaucanidrāmātsaryāgamyāgamanalolatāḥ ||
asatyabhāṣaṇaṃ cāpi kuryād dhi tāmase madaḥ ||209||

Suśrutasaṃhitā Cikitsāsthāna 24.90

na rājadviṣṭaparuṣapaiśunyānṛtāni vadet, na devabrāhmaṇapitṛparivādāṃś ca, na narendradviṣṭonmattapatitakṣudranīcān upāsīta ||90||

Carakasaṃhitā Śārīrasthāna 2.46

naro hitāhāravihārasevī samīkṣya kārī viṣayeṣv asaktaḥ |
dātā samaḥ satyaparaḥ kṣamāvān āptopasevī ca bhavaty arogaḥ ||46||

Aṣṭāṅgahṛdayasaṃhitā Śārīrasthāna 3.120

dānaśīladayāsatyabrahmacaryakṛtajñatāḥ |
rasāyanāni maitrī ca puṇyāyurvṛddhikṛd gaṇaḥ ||120||

Carakasaṃhitā Sūtrasthāna 7.26–30

imāṃs tu dhārayed vegān hitārthī pretya ceha ca |
sāhasānām aśastānāṃ manovākkāyakarmaṇām ||26||
lobhaśokabhayakrodhamānavegān vidhārayet |
nairlajjyerṣyātirāgāṇām abhidhyāyāś ca buddhimān ||27||
paruṣasyātimātrasya sūcakasyānṛtasya ca |
vākyasyākālayuktasya dhārayed vegam utthitam ||28||
dehapravṛttir yā kācid vidyate parapīḍayā |
strībhogasteyahiṃsādyā tasyā vegān vidhārayet ||29||
puṇyaśabdo vipāpatvān manovākkāyakarmaṇām |
dharmārthakāmān puruṣaḥ sukhī bhuṅkte cinoti ca ||30||

Ensuring Patient Compliance

Carakasaṃhitā Cikitsāsthāna 8.149–157

śuṣyatāṃ kṣīṇamāṃsānāṃ kalpitāni vidhānavit |
dadyān māṃsādamāṃsāni bṛṃhaṇāni viśeṣataḥ ||149||
śoṣiṇe bārhiṇaṃ dadyād barhiśabdena cāparān|
gṛdhrān ulūkāṃś cāṣāṃś ca vidhivat sūpakalpitān ||150||
kākās tittiriśabdena varmiśabdena coragān |
bhṛṣṭān matsyāntraśabdena dadyād gaṇḍūpadān api ||151||
lopākān sthūlanakulān biḍālāṃś copakalpitān |
śṛgālaśāvāṃś ca bhiṣak śaśaśabdena dāpayet ||152||
siṃhān ṛkṣāṃs tarakṣūṃś ca vyāghrān evaṃvidhāṃs tathā |
māṃsādān mṛgaśabdena dadyān māṃsābhivṛddhaye ||153||
gajakhaḍgituraṅgāṇāṃ veśavārīkṛtaṃ bhiṣak|
dadyān mahiṣaśabdena māṃsaṃ māṃsābhivṛddhaye ||154||
māṃsenopacitāṅgānāṃ māṃsaṃ māṃsakaraṃ param |
tīkṣṇoṣṇalāghavāc chastaṃ viśeṣān mṛgapakṣiṇām ||155||
māṃsāni yāny anabhyāsād aniṣṭāni prayojayet |
teṣūpadhā sukhaṃ bhoktuṃ tathā śakyāni tāni hi ||156||
jānañ jugupsan naivādyāj jagdhaṃ vā punar ullikhet |
tasmāc chadmopasiddhāni māṃsāny etāni dāpayet ||157||

Aṣṭāṅgahṛdayasaṃhitā Cikitsāsthāna 5.7

gṛdhrabhāsakharoṣṭraṃ ca hitaṃ chadmopasaṃhitam |
jñātaṃ jugupsitaṃ tad dhi chardiṣe na balaujase ||7||

Suśrutasaṃhitā Uttaratantra 41.35

kākān ulūkān nakulān biḍālān gaṇḍūpadān vyālabileśayākhūn ||
gṛdhrāṃś ca dadyād vividhaiḥ pravādaiḥ sasaindhavān sarṣapatailabhṛṣṭān ||35||

Suśrutasaṃhitā Cikitsāsthāna 1.82cd–83ab

māṃsāśināṃ ca māṃsāni bhakṣayed vidhivan naraḥ ||82cd||
viśuddhamanasas tasya māṃsaṃ māṃsena vardhate ||

Deception as a Therapeutic Tool

Carakasaṃhitā Cikitsāsthāna 9.79–84

āśvāsayet suhṛd vā taṃ vākyair dharmārthasaṃhitaiḥ |
brūyād iṣṭavināśaṃ vā darśayed adbhutāni vā ||79||
baddhaṃ sarṣapatailāktaṃ nyased vottānam ātape |
kapikacchvāthavā taptair lohatailajalaiḥ spṛśet ||80||
kaśābhis tāḍayitvā vā subaddhaṃ vijane gṛhe |
rundhyāc ceto hi vibhrāntaṃ vrajaty asya tathā śamam ||81||

sarpeṇoddhṛtadaṃṣṭreṇa dāntaiḥ siṃhair gajaiś ca tam |
trāsayec chastrahastair vā taskaraiḥ śatrubhis tathā ||82||
athavā rājapuruṣā bahir nītvā susaṃyatam |
trāsayeyur vadhenainaṃ tarjayanto nṛpājñayā ||83||
dehaduḥkhabhayebhyo hi paraṃ prāṇabhayaṃ smṛtam |
tena yāti śamaṃ tasya sarvato 'pi plutaṃ manaḥ ||84||

Suśrutasaṃhitā Uttaratantra 62.17–21b

darśayed adbhutāny asya, vaden nāśaṃ priyasya vā ||
bhīmākārair narair nāgair dāntair vyālaiś ca nirviṣaiḥ ||17||
bhīṣayet saṃyataṃ pāśaiḥ kaśābhir vātha tāḍayet |
yantrayitvā suguptaṃ vā trāsayet taṃ tṛṇāgninā ||18||
jalena tarjayed vāpi rajjughātair vibhāvayet |
balavāṃś cāpi saṃrakṣet jale 'ntaḥ parivāsayet ||19||
pratuded ārayā cainaṃ marmāghātaṃ vivarjayet |
veśmano 'ntaḥ praviśyainaṃ rakṣaṃs tad veśma dīpayet ||20||
sāpidhāne jaratkūpe satataṃ vā nivāsayet |

Notes

1. Excellent descriptions of some of the fundamental ayurvedic principles that recur in most ayurvedic works can be found in Jolly (1994 [1951]); Filliozat (1964); Wujastyk (2003), Mazars (1995), Basham (1998 [1976]), and in the appendix of Das (2003).
2. See also the German original of Jolly's book, *Medicin*, which dates to 1901. See also Liétard (1897, reprinted in Roşu 1989, 221–233) and Menon and Haberman (1970) for comparisons between the Hippocratic Oath and the teacher's speech at the medical student's initiation in the *Carakasaṃhitā* (Vi.8.13).
3. See Jolly (1994 [1951], 22–23) for a brief overview of analogies between Indian and Greek medicine.
4. On the "brahmanization" of Indian medicine, see Zysk 1998 [1991].
5. See also Lal 2005, 27–79, for the "history of ahistoricity" in India.
6. See chapter 2.
7. Preisendanz's forthcoming article "Medicine and Brahminical Orthodoxy in Ancient India: On Some Ritual Elements in the *Carakasaṃhitā*" is based on preliminary studies presented at the World Sanskrit Conference in Kyoto in September 2009.
8. Ainslie specifically mentioned Sonnerat's *Voyage to the East Indies*, which stated that "the Indians are mostly all pretenders to some knowledge of medicine; that there is not one physician amongst them more learned than another; that they are generally individuals who have been washermen, weavers, or blacksmiths, but a few months before; and, to crown all, that they administer few remedies inwardly, and make little use of ointments or cataplasms." See Ainslie 1813, 64. The same passage is reprinted in Ainslie 1826, xxviii–xxx. This seems to have been a contentious issue. See, for example, Heyne (1814, 125), who noted that it "is common in India to hear the native physicians represented by some Europeans as a set of ignorant cheats, and extolled by others as miracles of knowledge and wisdom." Heyne himself was of the opinion that most Indian physicians were indeed cheats and quacks, and that only a small number of skilled and knowledgeable physicians were to be found among them. On the subject of the ayurvedic works, Heyne took the stand that they were "neither

to be regarded as miraculous productions of wisdom, nor as repositories of nonsense."

9. Ibid.
10. Ibid.
11. I.e., "Agastya's five hundred verses on medicine." I would like to thank Dr. R. Weiss for helping me to translate the title of the Tamil text. In chapter 2, Ainslie lists a number of Tamil medical works, noting that his source for this list was procured for him by a Dr. M. Christy, from "a learned Brahmin belonging to the great pagoda at Madura." See Ainslie 1826, 504.
12. See As.Sū.2.7–20 on a physician's professional conduct.
13. See Wilson 1823, 350–357.
14. Wise claimed to have compared the medical works of Caraka and Suśruta, and to have compiled commentaries, rejecting "some portions as worthless" while retaining "all such parts as appeared peculiar in theory, or important in practice," and even restoring passages "altered by the carelessness or ignorance of compilers or of commentators." See Wise 1845, xviii–xix. Wise noted that he received assistance from pandits to undertake this work, specifically naming "Abhaycharan Tarkapanchanan, superintendent of the Bengali department of the College of Muhammad Mohsem, Hoogly," and "Madhusudan Gupta, Lecturer of anatomy to the Medical College, Calcutta." The latter scholar was perhaps most famous for having been the first Indian known to have undertaken a dissection in 1836. See Arnold 1993, 6, and Magner 1997, 150.
15. See Preisendanz (2007, 636) for an identification of the passages in the medical works that underlie Wise's study.
16. In his bibliography, Sinh Jee listed an impressive number of Sanskrit medical works. However, this list is perhaps better understood as a list of medical works known to Sinh Jee than as references to works actually cited or paraphrased in his book. There is some reason to believe that Sinh Jee's book was actually authored by Jīvarāma Kālidāsa Shastri, the Rājavaidya ("King's physician") at the court of Gondal, where Sinh Jee was Mahārāja. Personal communication between Dominik Wujastyk and Ghanashyamji (Shastri's son) in 1992 at the Rasashāstra Oushadhālaya in Gondal, Gujarat.
17. See the reprint of these essays in Roşu 1989. The case of the essay entitled "Suşruta" is puzzling, since the article is reproduced in Roşu's anthology, but not listed in his bibliography of Liétard's works. In dating this article, I follow an entry found in Copac (www.copac.ac.uk), which also has a question mark behind the date. The Copac entry refers to an entry from the Wellcome Library for the History and Understanding of Medicine.
18. His main references are to the *Mānavadharmaśāstra* and to the *Yājñavalkyasmṛti*. See Cordier 1989, 505.
19. See Zimmer 1948, 75–95.
20. See Basham 1967, 498–500.

21. On this topic, see chapter 6.
22. See Chattopadhyaya 1977, 58. Dominik Wujastyk, in his article "Medicine and Dharma" came to a similar conclusion, i.e., that a physician's moral choices are guided by medical expedience. See Wujastyk 2004b, 836.
23. See also my discussion of this passage in the last section of chapter 2.
24. See Desai 1995.
25. See Mazars 1995, 92–104.
26. See Jonsen 2000, 27–43.
27. See the preface, "From the Author's Desk," in Athavale and Athavale 2003, x.
28. For example, the authors claim that education was free, enabling the rich as well as the poor to have a career of their choice. See Athavale and Athavale 2003, 13–14. The *Carakasaṃhitā* mentions the teacher's fee (*gurvartha*) but does not specify how much this is or what it consists of. While this allows for the speculation that a poor student may not have had to pay much, it does not provide safe grounds for the Athavales' assertion of free education for all.
29. See Crawford 2003, 51–55.
30. Here, Crawford used Haberman's and Menon's translation.
31. See Crawford 2003, 197.
32. The declaration of Geneva, for example, was meant to be an update of the Hippocratic Oath.
33. However, there has been a steady interest from pharmacists, pharmacologists, and the pharmacological industry in the *materia medica* of ayurvedic works that has resulted in a large number of scientific publications on the medical and cosmetic uses of South Asian plants. This interest has now intensified after recent debates about green imperialism and biopiracy. See, for example, Banerjee 1995 and Bode 2008.
34. See, for example, Chattopadhyaya (1977, 19) who gives the term *vṛddhatrayī*—the "old threesome," instead of *bṛhattrayī* for the *Carakasaṃhitā*, the *Suśruta-saṃhitā*, and the *Aṣṭāṅgasaṃgraha*.
35. See Wujastyk 2003, 3–5.
36. See Meulenbeld (1999–2002, IA, 105–115) for a more detailed discussion of the dating of the *Carakasaṃhitā*.
37. See Wujastyk 2003, 63–64.
38. See Meulenbeld (1999–2002, IA, 342–352) for a detailed survey of the discussions on the different layers of the *Suśrutasaṃhitā*, and the dating of these.
39. See Meulenbeld 1999–2002, IA, 631–635 .
40. See Meulenbeld (1999–2002, IA, 613–626) for a discussion of the date of the *Aṣṭāṅgasaṃgraha*.
41. This is also true for the *Kāśyapasaṃhitā*, and the *Bhelasaṃhitā*. Mādhava's authorship of the *Mādhavanidāna* is less contentious, as is Śārṅgadhara's of the *Śārṅgadharasaṃhitā* and Bhāvamiśra's of the *Bhāvaprakāśa*.

42. It can, however, be difficult to make a strong case for the popularity of a text based on the numbers of manuscript copies available to us today for a number of reasons. The first is that the numbers of manuscript copies may be difficult to determine, since many manuscripts may have been lost with time. Then, those that are still preserved may not have been catalogued. Note, for example, that the *New Catalogus Catalogorum* lists about 110 manuscripts of the *Carakasaṃhitā* (or parts of it), while about 150 manuscripts are used for the critical edition of the *Carakasaṃhitā* in the Vienna project. On the other hand, if a great number of manuscripts does exist, as in the case of the *Aṣṭāṅgahṛdayasaṃhitā*, then we can be sure of a text's importance.
43. See Meulenbeld 1999–2002, vol. IA, 180–200.
44. See Meulenbeld 1999–2002, vol. IA, 372–389.
45. See Meulenbeld 1999–2002, vol. IA, 661–685.
46. See Meulenbeld 1999–2002, vol. IA, 656.
47. See Meulenbeld 1999–2002, vol. IIA, 61.
48. See Meulenbeld 1999–2002, vol. IIA, 65–67. Though of great importance to the ayurvedic tradition, the *Mādhavanidāna* yields little material on medical ethics, and is therefore of less interest to this study than the other treatises.
49. See Meulenbeld 1999–2002, vol. IIA, 207–210.
50. See Wujastyk 2003, 255.
51. See Meulenbeld 1999–2002, vol. IIA, 242.
52. The bad state of the manuscripts is the reason why in references to the second chapter of the Kāśyapasaṃhitā's Vimānasthāna (Kāś.Vi.) a question mark in parentheses is placed behind the chapter number: there may have been further preceding chapters.
53. See Meulenbeld 1999–2002, IA, 378.
54. See Meulenbeld 1999–2002, 669–674.
55. See Meulenbeld 1999–2002, IIA, 207–210.
56. See As.Sū.2.7 and also Ca.Sū.29.8, which refers to quacks as "thorns" (*kaṇṭaka*) in parallel to Kauṭilya's usage in K.A.4.1.56.
57. See Olivelle 2005, xvi.
58. Olivelle (1999, xxv–xxxiv) notes that there is no straightforward answer to the questions who wrote these works and when they were written. Even their relative chronology to each other is uncertain. However, he proposes that the youngest of the texts is that by Vasiṣṭha, preceded by the older parts of Baudhāyana's text; that Āpastamba is older than Gautama, and probably even older than the text of the early parts of Baudhāyana; and that Gautama is also older than even the earlier parts of Baudhāyana. Olivelle tentatively places the earlier works between the beginning of the third to the middle of the second century BCE, and Vasiṣṭha somewhat later.
59. FWF (Austrian Science Fund) project nos. P 14451-G03 (preliminary research), P 17300-G03 ("Philosophy and Medicine in Early Classical India

I"), and now P 19866-G15 ("Philosophy and Medicine in Early Classical India II"). The critical edition will be published with the Österreichische Akademie der Wissenschaften. For further information on the project, see www.istb.univie.ac.at/caraka/.

60. See http://indology.info/email/members/setzer/.
61. See Wujastyk (2003, xxxv–xxxviii) on the problems one faces in trying to identify ayurvedic plants.
62. Web site consulted in March 2009.
63. I have chosen the translation "pillar" for *pāda*, instead of, for example, "part" or "fourth," in order to convey the sense that each part of the quartet is a means of support without which medicine could not stand.
64. See Ca.Sū.9, Su.Sū.34.15cd–24, Ah.Sū.1.27–29, As.Sū.2.21–25ab, Kāś.Sū.26.3–11, Bhel.Sū.9. There is a passing mention of the four pillars in Mādh.5.39, with a lengthy commentary on it in Vācaspati's commentary, the Ātaṅkadarpaṇa. A good translation of this passage in Vācaspati's commentary is found in Meulenbeld 2008, 247, which gives Su.Sū.34.15cd–16ab and 19cd–24 as its source.
65. I read "humor" instead of "bodily tissues" or "bodily elements" for "*dhātu*" here, following H. Scharfe's study of the use of the terms *dhātu* and *doṣa* in the *Carakasaṃhitā*, in which Scharfe concludes: "To sum up: the older parts of the Caraka-saṃhitā consider wind, bile, and phlegm in their natural state as elements [dhātu] and only in their riled condition as faults [doṣa]. Health is a balance of the elements [dhātu]" (Scharfe, 1999, 624). However, Cakrapāṇidatta defines *dhātu* as an umbrella term for the humors (i.e., *vāta*, *pitta*, and *kapha*), the bodily tissues (beginning with chyle, *rasa*), and the psychological elements (beginning with passion, *rajas*): *dhātavo vātādayo rasādayaś ca tathā rajaḥprabhṛtayaś ca*. See also Maas (2009, 137–138) for lists of text passages in the *Carakasaṃhitā* that define the term *dhātu*. Quite often, these definitions show *dhātu* to be an umbrella term for the bodily elements (flesh, blood, bone, etc.) as well as the humors (wind, bile, phlegm), as well as for other bodily substances. Therefore, this verse may equally refer to an imbalance of all bodily substances. However, Maas (2009, 136) also argues that "the three elements wind, phlegm and bile are most important among the listed bodily constituents, since their ratio is stressed as the decisive factor for health and disease." I agree with this assessment, and therefore interpret *dhātu* here as "humor."
66. Cakrapāṇidatta explains that they are praised in connection with certain qualities that are laid out in the following sentences.
67. This translation of *tatrayogyatva* does not give a correlation of *tatra*, "in that case," "there." Cakrapāṇidatta explains *tatra* to refer to an illness: *tatra pratikartavye vyādhau yogatvaṃ tatrayogatvam*—"'tatrayogatva' means suitability in the case of an illness that is to be counteracted." Suitability therefore refers to the correct choice of medicine for an illness.

68. I.e., that a plant can be used in different ways: as a juice, or a paste, etc. Cakrapāṇidatta explains that it can be necessary to offer patients alternatives, since some people dislike juices, others dislike pastes, etc. He also adds that for some illnesses specific preparations are required, such as astringent juice (*kaṣāya*) for fevers.
69. I understand the term *saṃpad* to mean "excellent quality" here, implying the perfection and completeness of the plants' potency and other properties. In this, I follow Cakrapāṇidatta's interpretation: "*saṃpad iti krimisalilādyanupahatatvena rasādisaṃpat*," "'Excellent quality' means excellent quality in taste, etc., because of being undamaged by worms or water, etc." Taste (*rasa*) is one of four standard classifications of the properties (*guṇa*) of a medicinal plant. The other three are potency (*vīrya*), the taste of food after digestion (*vipāka*), and specific action (*prabhāva*). The latter is used to explain the effect of a drug that does not follow from its taste, potency, or postdigestive taste. This is laid out in Ca.Sū.26. See also Meulenbeld's reflections on these properties as basic concepts of Indian pharmacology (Meulenbeld, 1987). Cakrapāṇidatta's explanation that something is *saṃpad* because it is unimpaired, points to the meaning of *saṃpad* in the sense of "completeness." Bodewitz (2003, 239), summarizing Wezler's interpretation of *saṃpad* (see Wezler 2003), writes that "the actual presence of all qualities which a particular class of entities or things can theoretically have, in such an entity or thing makes it 'perfect.'" Bodewitz generally disagrees with Wezler's interpretation of *saṃpad* (in the K.A.), preferring "success" instead. The latter meaning cannot, however, be applied to the passage here.
70. Cakrapāṇidatta adds the following explanations: *vijñātā auṣadhasya | śāsitā paricārakasya—evam kurv evaṃ mā kurv iti | yoktā āturasya*, "One who knows about medicines, who instructs the attendant with the words do it like this, don't do it like that, who applies effort to the patient."
71. Cakrapāṇidatta interprets *nāvahanti guṇaṃ* as "not effecting cure," glossing *nāvahanti* ("they do not lead towards") with *na niṣpādayanti* ("they do not effect"), and *guṇa* ("good quality") with *sādhya* ("cure").
72. I.e., like a mirage.
73. The concept of someone's life being fixed, i.e., predetermined, is discussed in Ca.Vi.3.28–36, followed by a pertinent discussion on timely and untimely death in Vi.3.37–38. See Wujastyk 2003, 44–47, for a translation of these sections. According to these passages, life span is determined by two factors: the influences of fate (*daiva*) and human action (*puruṣakāra*). "Fate" represents actions done in previous lives that bear on the present life. It is the same idea as the concept of *karma*, according to which we reap the fruits of our actions in the next life. Human effort, on the other hand, concerns any action taken in this life, including lifestyle choices and the application of medical treatments. At the same time, a certain life expectancy is presupposed, both in the sense

that we can reasonably expect a number of years to live and that we must die. Whether someone's life expectancy is fulfilled depends on the aforementioned factors. Bad actions in previous lives may have such strong effect that they cannot be canceled out by any action in this life. Conversely, good actions done in previous lives may bear positively on negative situations in this life. Caraka proposes varying grades of strength (strong, medium, or weak) in these influences, suggesting that they take effect, supersede each other, or cancel each other out depending on their relative grade to each other. It would take strong human action to undo a medium or a weak fate. But if fate is strong, it cannot be outdone by weak or medium action. Therefore, it follows that the actions of persons believing themselves to be physicians must be categorized as weak or medium, so that they cannot counteract the positive, strong fate at work in the lucky patient, who thus survives their attentions.

74. Wezler (1984, 307–312) referred to this verse, suggesting that it may be related to the concept of four divisions that, according to the *Yogabhāṣya* (the commentary part of the *Yogaśāstra*) on *Yogasūtra* 2.15, are found in a *cikitsāśāstra*. The latter may either denote a particular work on medicine (that is, however, unknown to us) or may be a reference to medical science. The four divisions ascribed to the *cikitsāśāstra* are "*rogo rogahetur ārogyaṃ bhaiśajyam,*" "illness, the cause of illness, health, and medicine." They are paralleled by the Yoga concepts of "*saṃsāraḥ saṃsārahetur mokṣo mokṣopāya,*" "worldly existence, the cause of worldly existence, spiritual emancipation, the means to spiritual emancipation." Wezler concludes that Caraka's verse is similar in content to the purported division of the *cikitsāśāstra* and to the Four Noble Truths—(i.e., the nature of suffering (Skt. *duḥkha*, Pāli *dukkha*), its origin (Skt. *samudaya*), its cessation (Skt./Pāli *nirodha*) and the path leading to its cessation (Skt. *nirodhagāminī pratipad*, Pāli *nirodhagāminī paṭipada*))—but that the fourfold division seems not to have been of any importance to medicine as represented by the medical classics. Wezler also stressed that one cannot prove an actual connection between the Four Noble Truths and the fourfold division of a *cikitsāśāstra*.
75. Cakrapāṇidatta suggests *āśraya* to mean having recourse to a good teacher.
76. Cakrapāṇidatta interprets *śāstra* as "the mind that has undergone study of the science" (*śāstrābhyāsakṛtā mati*).
77. I understand "natural state" to mean health. In medical literature, *prakṛti* in relation to humans usually refers to a person's constitution or temperament, i.e., the physical and mental setup that is governed by the relative amounts of humors (wind, *vāta*, bile, *pitta*, and phlegm, *kapha*) in someone's body. A person can be defined as *vātala*, *pittala*, and *kaphala*, according to whichever humor is predominantly present in his body. Caraka discusses this in Vi.6.13–19 and points out a divergence in opinion between different schools of thought. The first (see Ca.Vi.6.13) defines health (*ārogya*) as subject to a perfect balance of

the three humors, i.e., that there are equal amounts of the humoral substances in the body. Health is then declared to be a person's natural or normal state (*prakṛti*). This natural state thus only refers to the condition of someone whose humors are in complete balance, and who therefore has no predominance of one of the three humors. By contrast, the second school of thought maintains that having a greater quantity of one of the humors can be part of one's nature (see Ca.Vi.6.15–19) and does not necessarily make a person ill. The predominance merely effects the person in the form of a specific sensitivity to foods, activities, etc. that would aggravate or accumulate the predominant humor in his body. According to this interpretation, health is not subject to an equal measure of humors but to a relative balance of the humors, and *prakṛti* signifies someone's individual natural state. Just as in the first school of thought, however, the natural state of a person is health: *prakṛti* equals *ārogya*.
However, Cakrapāṇidatta suggests a rather different meaning for *prakṛtistha*: "approaching death." Cakrapāṇidatta argues: "*prakṛtir iha maraṇaṃ, prakṛtir ucyate svabhāvaḥ; tathā—"idam (read ayam) asmān muhūrtāt ... svabhāvam āpatsyate*" (Ca.Sū.30.25), maraṇam ity arthaḥ; maraṇasamīpagatatvād ucyate 'prakṛtisthe' iti. tasminn upekṣā kartavyā; na tatra bheṣajadānādi kartavyaṃ, yaśohānyādibhayāt": " 'Natural condition' [*prakṛti*] here means 'dying', '*prakṛti*' is called 'natural state'; thus "He, from this moment on . . . will hasten toward his natural state," i.e., to death; from the state of having come close to death, it is called 'being in a natural state.' In this case, indifference is necessary; under this circumstance, medicine should not be administered, etc., for fear of damaging one's reputation." Francis Zimmermann draws attention to the same passages in his online reflections "L'amitié pour tous les êtres, la compassion pour les malades," at http://ehess.philosophindia.fr/inde/36/ (consulted in April 2008) Cakrapāṇidatta's argument is based on equating *prakṛti* with *svabhāva*, which also means "natural state," etc. In Ca.Sū.30.25, the passage that Cakrapāṇidatta partially quotes, *svabhāva* is stated to have the same meaning as *pravṛtter uparama* (cessation of activity), *maraṇa* (death), *anityatā* (noneternalness) and *nirodha* (annihilation). Having defined *prakṛti* as a synonym to *svabhāva* therefore allows Cakrapāṇidatta to make the leap to interpreting *prakṛti* as "death" and *prakṛtistha* as "approaching death." However, "approaching" (following Cakrapāṇidatta's *samīpagata*) hardly is an accurate rendering of *stha*. I find Cakrapāṇidatta's argument unconvincing, particularly given that Caraka himself does not make this connection but does define *prakṛti* as health at length. I therefore do not follow Cakrapāṇidatta's interpretation in this instance.

78. Ca.Sū.8.17 states this explicitly.
79. I count as overlap not only words that are repeated, such as *vidyā*, but also words that denote the same thing, as for example *dṛṣṭakarmatā*, *karmadarśana*, and *karmadṛṣṭi*.
80. Ca.Sū.9.20 and 25 are exceptions.

81. These are also called the *apramāṇa* (Pāli: *appamāṇa*). See Maithrimurthi 1999, 13–46.
82. See Woodward et al. 1986-92, V.299. Maithrimurthi (1999, 35–36) provides references to other sources on the *brahmavihāra,* both in the Pāli Canon, in other Buddhist sources, and in non-Buddhist sources.
83. See Maithrimurthi (1999, 187–214) on the *brahmavihāra* in the Visuddhimagga and the Abhidharmakośa.
84. For a list of similarities between the Pātañjala Yoga and various Buddhist doctrines, including the *brahmavihāra,* see de La Vallée Poussin (1936–37).
85. The *udgātṛ, hotṛ, brahman,* and *adhvaryu* are the different types of priests who officiate at Vedic sacrifices. The *hotṛ* ("sacrificer" or "summoner") invokes the gods at the sacrifice, reciting stanzas from the Ṛgveda (one of four canonical Vedic text compilations that form the basis of brahmanic religion). The *udgātṛ* ("chanter") chants the hymns of the Sāmaveda (the second of the Vedic canonical compilations). The *brahmin* who knows the Vedic compilations (i.e., Ṛg-, Sāma-, Yajur-, and Atharvaveda) supervises the sacrifice and corrects mistakes. Finally, the *adhvaryu* is responsible for preparing the setting for the sacrifice, i.e., preparing the ground, the altar, the fire, the sacrificial vessels, etc., while reciting stanzas from the Yajurveda. His role is therefore crucial to the execution of a sacrifice, which must be held in a certain setting with particular implements. For a description and discussion of the role of the Vedic compilations in brahmanic religion, see, for example, Staal 2008 or Hillebrandt 1897.
86. Ḍalhaṇa explains that the humors wind, etc., are understood as that by which the bodily elements (*dhātu*) and the waste products (*mala*), etc., are spoilt. He adds that "the removal of humors means to remove what is spoilt, and not to irritate that which is unspoilt" (*doṣaharaṃ duṣṭiṃ haraty, aduṣṭaṃ na ca kopayati*). In Su.Cik.33.3f., Suśruta explains that "diminished faults must be strengthened, riled [faults] calmed, increased [faults] removed, balanced [faults] protected: that is the authoritative doctrine. Most prominently, emetics and purgatives are used to remove faults" (Scharfe, 1999, 626). I do not agree with Scharfe's translation of *doṣa* as "fault," which does not fit the context of the passage and stands at odds with Suśruta's definition that *doṣas* are the root of the body (see Su.Sū.15.3). However, the image of increased *doṣas* that need to be removed fits the context of Su.Sū.34.23, which is why I have translated *doṣaghna* as "removing [excess] humors."
87. "This explains one of the most curious aspects of the medical treatises: the king is the most important of all patients, *the king is the patient par excellence,* because his state of health expresses the *artha* (well-being) of all his subjects" (Zimmermann, 1999 [1987], 181).
88. While it is certainly possible that an attendant's work could have been done by females—particularly in the case of female patients—I follow the medical

authors' conventional use of the masculine gender to describe attendants with my use of the masculine pronoun only.

89. Aruṇadatta explains *jñāpaka* with *nidānāvasthādīnām āvedakaḥ*, "who reports on the causes, his condition, etc."
90. Su.Sū.34.19.
91. See Ca.Sū.9.22.
92. The use of the term *saṃpad* here could be understood to mean "success" rather than "perfection," i.e., "by which success in medical treatment is arrived at." However, in the following paragraphs, *saṃpad* is connected with the qualities of medicines, attendants, and patients, and in none of these cases does the translation "success" (or "successful") quite fit. In those cases, I prefer the translation of *saṃpad* as "complete group/aggregate/assemblage" that Wezler (2003, 438ff.) proposes in cases (in the K.A.) where *saṃpad* follows an enumeration of decisive factors. I use "perfection," then, in the sense of "something that is complete."
93. Or "is a good teacher." In the absence of a commentary, it is difficult to decide whether Kaśyapa intended the physician to be connected to a good teacher or felt that it was a good physician's characteristic that he could teach well.
94. The additions in brackets reflect my interpretation rather than the literal meaning of the sentence.
95. This translation of *vaidyavidagdha* follows Cakrapāṇidatta's gloss of the term in his commentary on Ca.Si.2.5 (which Bhāvamiśra quotes here). Cakrapāṇidatta equates *vaidyavidagdha* with *vaidyamānin*, "One who thinks himself a physician." Also see Ḍalhaṇa on Su.Sū.10.8, where *vaidyavidagdha* also occurs. Ḍalhaṇa glosses it with *vaidyābhimānin*, "one who thinks of himself as a physician," and *pallavagrāhin*, "one whose knowledge is superficial."
96. I am not quite sure what is meant by *sajīvadiś*, "place/direction that has life." This sentence is a quotation from the *Śārṅgadharasaṃhitā* (Pūrv.3.12). In Ca.Ind.12.15., a chapter on the signs of a patient's imminent death, Caraka notes that if a messenger comes to the physician at a place or time that is connected to the disease (*vikārasāmānya*), then the physician should not treat the patient.
97. I.e., moist, cool, gentle. On the division of all substances into a dichotomy of *soma* and *agni*, cold/wet and hot/dry, as a fundamental principle of ayurvedic theory, see Wujastyk 2004a.
98. The term *pradīpta* here stands for *agneya*, hot and dry, as the opposite of *saumya*. See note 97.
99. See note 86.
100. Cakrapāṇidatta also places several of the terms that follow "knowledge" in Ca.Sū.9.21 (namely "reason," "understanding," "devotion," etc.) into a medical context: "*vitarkaḥ śāstramūla ūhāpohaḥ | vijñānaṃ śāstrāntarajñānaṃ, kiṃvā*

sahajaṃ viśuddhiṃ jñānam | tatparateha vyādhicikitsāyāṃ prayatnātiśayatvam | kriyā punaḥ punaś cikitsākaraṇam | matiḥ sahajaviśuddhimatiḥ | abhyāsaḥ karmābhyāsaḥ | siddhiḥ prāyaśo vyādhipraśamatvam | āśrayaḥ sadgurvāśraya ity arthaḥ": "'Reason,' the root of the science, means conjecture and refutation. 'Understanding' means knowledge of the treatise's contents, or innate perfect knowledge. 'Devotion' here means extreme diligence in the treatment of disorders. 'Action' again means performing medical treatment. 'Intelligence' means intelligence that is innate perfect knowledge. 'Practice' means practicing medical treatment. 'Success' generally means curing illnesses. 'Support' means the support of a good teacher."

101. Or "who are approaching death"; see note 77.
102. Suśruta's argument appears again in As.Sū.2.9cd-11ab. Verse 48 is quoted verbatim, and verse 49 is paraphrased, but verse 50 is not repeated.
103. Pollock 1985, 509–510. Pollock quotes K.A. 1.8.25 ("One who knows *śāstra* but is inexperienced will come to grief in practical application") as an example of Kauṭilya's attitude.
104. Ca.Sū.1.135. See below for the full passage.
105. See Pollock 1985 on the meanings encompassed by the term *śāstra*.
106. It should be noted, however, that this can also be translated as "a good teacher," i.e., that a physician should be a good teacher.
107. Parallel passages in the other medical treatises are Ca.Vi.8.9–14, Su.Sū.2.4–10, Kāś.Vi.2(?).3–6, and As.Sū.2.6–7a.
108. Translation of Ca.Sū.11.50–53 by Dominik Wujastyk (2003, 33).
109. A word search of the expression *bhiṣaṅmānin* in the electronic texts of the medical treatises available to me (i.e., the *Carakasaṃhitā*, *Suśrutasaṃhitā*, *Aṣṭāṅgahṛdayasaṃhitā*, *Aṣṭāṅgasaṃgraha*, *Śārṅgadharasaṃhitā*, and *Bhāvaprakāśa*) only brought up this passage. Its synonym *vaidyamānin* occurs four times in the same sources, but only once to denote someone acting as a physician (in Ca.Sū.16.4). The other three instances ascribe the characteristic of thinking themselves a physician to patients who are best to be avoided by the physician (see Ca.Vi.3.45, Ah.Sū.1.35, and As.Sū.2.19, respectively).
110. This passage reads: "There are indeed two kinds of physician, Sir Agniveśa. Some are savers of life and destroyers of disease, others are savers of disease and destroyers of life."
111. I.e., the ten seats of vital breath, which are described in the previous sentence.
112. Ca.Sū.29.4.
113. Wujastyk 2003, 30. Addition in brackets mine.
114. This is the beginning of Ca.Sū.29.7.
115. Not belonging to a disreputable family is mentioned by Kaśyapa as a characteristic of the perfect attendant, but not of the physician.
116. Su.Sū.2.3. The word used is *anvaya* ("family").
117. *tadvidyakulaja*, "born into a family of experts."

118. Meulenbeld (1999–2002, 26) makes note of this in his summary of Ca.Sū.29. The exceptions are chapters 6, "On What Should be Eaten," 15, "On Preparing Medicines," and 16, "On the Skilful Physician," which get no mention. However, the contents of the latter two may be understood to be summarized briefly by "inducing sweating, emesis, and purging." Chapters 25–28 are not sharply differentiated, though generally covered in the summary. Of the contents of Ca.Sū.11 only the three desires get listed, omitting the other groups of threes (subpillars, strength, causes of disorders, types of diseases, passages of diseases, types of therapy, etc.).
119. See Ca.Sū.9.15–17, p. 28.
120. See Su.Sū.25.41.
121. Ca.Sū.9.15. See "The Four Pillars of Medicine According to Caraka" earlier.
122. Su.Sū.25.41 and 32. See also Ca.Sū.1.126–131: "Through [proper] application even a sharp poison becomes an excellent medicine. A wrongly applied medicine, on the other hand, turns into a sharp poison. (126) Therefore a sensible person wishing to live and to be healthy should not take any medicine administered by a physician who is ignorant of the proper application [of medicines]. (127) Indra's thunderbolt, even if it has fallen onto [someone's] head, may spare [him], but a medicine approved by one who is ignorant, will not spare a patient. (128) One who, thinking himself learned, gives medicines without discernment to an afflicted, bedridden, and trusting patient (129): a person would fall into hell just by talking with him who has abandoned righteousness, who is evil, death personified, and malicious: (130) It is better to drink a decoction of snake poison, or of copper, or to imbibe red-hot iron-balls. (131)." See also As.Sū.2.20: "A person who wishes to live, even though he is ill, [should avoid] those physicians who have abandoned the good qualities mentioned before who sell their treatments and who truly precede death."
123. See "The Patient" earlier on this subject.
124. See also my discussion above of this category.
125. Wujastyk 2003, 33.
126. Synopses of this passage are found in Basham 1998 [1976], 30, Jolly 1994 [1951], 26, and Valiathan 2003, 144–145.
127. The translation in brackets adds the part omitted in Dominik Wujastyk's translation.
128. Translation by Dominik Wujastyk (1993, 762) from "Attired in doctor's outfits" to "the right attitude."
129. This etiquette is discussed in detail in chapter 20.
130. Bhāv.Pūrv.6.52. See "The Components of Treatment According to Bhāvamiśra" earlier. In later ayurvedic mythology, Dhanvantari is the god of healing. See also Meulenbeld 1999–2002, vol. IA, 358–361.
131. See chapter 2.
132. Basham 1998 [1976], 30.

133. See chapter 5 in regard to the inscription on the Viṣṇu temple of Veṅkateśa-Perumāḷ at Tirumukkūḍal from about the ninth century that records salaries for medical personnel who staffed a hospital (*āturaśālā*).
134. Siegel's sources include Śyāmilaka's *Pādatāḍitaka* (c. 5th century), Mahendravikramavarman's *Bhagavadajjukīya* (c. 7th century), Kṣemendra's *Deśopadeśa*, *Kalāvilāsa*, and *Narmamālā* (all c. early 11th century), Śaṅkhadhara's *Laṭakamelaka* (c. 12th century), Jagadīśvara Bhaṭṭācārya's *Hāsyārṇavaprahasana* (c. 14th century), Nīlakaṇṭha Dīkṣita's *Kaliviḍambana* (16th–17th century), Veṅkaṭādhvarin's *Viśvaguṇādarśacampū* (17th century), Lakṣmana Māṇikyadeva's *Kautukaratnākara* (c. 17th century) and the *Subhāṣitaratnabhaṇḍāgāra* (19th century).
135. This is perhaps the greatest difference between the Indian classical medical texts and the ancient Greek ones, which give many accounts of particular cases to draw a general theory of medicine. See, for example, Nutton (2004, 89) who describes the selection and organization of case histories in *Epidemics* of the Hippocratic corpus according to their usefulness for prognosis. The Buddhist Pāli Canon gives case histories, which Zysk (2000, 84–116, 120–127) discusses. The stories in the Buddhist monastic code serve as guidelines to "the permissable treatments that follow the rules pertaining to materia medica" and also "afforded monks and nuns a case-by-case instruction for the care of the sick" (Zysk, 2000, 84). The difference between this use of case histories and that of the Greek is that the cases described in the Canon are not used to form a general theory of medicine.
136. Kaśyapa's list of characteristics follows the heading "Perfection in a patient is . . ." (rather than "The perfect patient is . . ."), which does not pinpoint the gender of the patient. He uses the same phrasing for the attendant, again leaving open the option that the attendant may be female. Only his physician is clearly masculine. However, for the purpose of brevity, I will use the masculine pronoun for Kaśyapa's patient unless the feminine gender is used in the Sanskrit text.
137. Translation by Zysk 2000, 41, of *Mahāvagga* 8.26.6. Emphasis mine.
138. Wujastyk 2003, 88.
139. Wujastyk 2003, 89. Additions in brackets mine. See also "The *Suśrutasaṃhitā* on physicians' professional conduct" in chapter 2.
140. Kāś.Sū.26.8.
141. See Wujastyk (2003, 15–17) for a translation of the relevant passage of the *Carakasaṃhitā* describing the suppression of natural urges such as sneezing etc. as detrimental to one's health.
142. Suśruta names priests among those who are difficult to treat (Sū.10.8), and his commentator Ḍalhaṇa explains this to be due to their frequent ritual bathing. See Wujastyk 2003, 89.
143. Ah.Śā.6.72b–73ab.
144. Su.Sū.2.8.

145. See Su.Sū.10.8: "Even curable diseases can become extremely hard to treat in the following types: priests, kings, women, children, old people, scared people, royal servants, frauds, weak people, physicians, sly people, people who hide their ailments, poor people, misers, angry people, those who have no self-control, and those with no one to look after their interests. Watching out for this sort of thing, he who practices medicine achieves virtue, prosperity, enjoyment and fame" (Wujastyk, 2003, 90). Wujastyk separates *vaidya* and *vidagdha* into "physicians" and "sly people" here. However, Ḍalhaṇa's commentary glosses *vaidyavidagdha* as a compound with *vaidyābhimānin*, "one who fancies himself a physician," i.e., a quack. The term *vaidyavidagdha* also appears in Ca.Si.2.5, where it is also glossed as *vaidyamānin*, "one who believes himself a physician," by Cakrapāṇidatta. Also see note 95.
146. See Wujastyk 2003, 90.
147. Ca.Vi.3.45. See "The Patient" in chapter 1.
148. "*Adhanasyānupakaraṇatvena na cikitsā pāryate kartum ity arthaḥ*," Medical treatment cannot be done for a poor person, because of his not being furnished with equipment.
149. Ca.Cik.1.54–55. See appendix E for the Sanskrit text.
150. See Zimmermann 1999 [1987], 181.
151. See Su.Sū.10.8.
152. See Meulenbeld 1999–2002, 487.
153. "*te hi pramādaparigatā duḥkhāsahiṣṇavaś ca svayam apy apathyarucayaḥ*," As.Sū.8.3, middle part.
154. Su.Sū.34.10cd–12ab.
155. Ah.Sū.1.34–35ab gives "A physician should avoid patients who are despised by kings, who are their enemies, and hostile, those that are unequipped, inattentive, not compliant or very old, (34) those patients that are violent, afflicted by sorrow, cowardly, ungrateful, and who think themselves physicians." See "The *Aṣṭāṅgasaṃgraha* on Physicians' Professional Conduct," for As.Sū.2.18–19, in chapter 2.
156. "*caṇḍādiṣu pravṛttir bheṣajasyāśakyatvān niṣidhyate; kṛtaghnādiṣu cādharmavaśād eva bheṣajaṃ na sidhyati, pratyutādhārmikapratikriyayā 'dharma eva bhavatīti nivṛttir vidhīyate*," Cakrapāṇidatta on Siddhisthāna 2.4–6.
157. Grief (*śoka*) is regarded as an urge that should be suppressed by Caraka. In Sū.7.27, he juxtaposes grief with greed, fear, anger, conceit, shamelessness, envy, obsession, and longing: "*Lobhaśokabhayakrodhamānavegān vidhārayet nairlajjyerṣyātirāgāṇām abhidhyāyāś ca buddhimān*," "A wise person should check the urges of greed, grief, fear, anger, and conceit, as well as those of shamelessness, envy, obsession, and longing." This places the grieving person into the same category as the violent, cowardly, ungrateful, and inconsiderate persons.

158. See page 165 for the Sanskrit text of this passage.
159. See Ca.Sū.8.32–33.
160. Ca.Sū.9.8.
161. See Su.Sū.34.24, Ah.Sū. 1.29, and As.Sū.2.25, respectively.
162. Kāś.Sū.26.7.
163. Translation by Dominik Wujastyk (2003, 132). Addition in brackets mine.
164. Translation by Zysk (2000, 41) of *Mahāvagga* 8.26.3.
165. Translation by Zysk (2000, 42) of *Mahāvagga* 8.26.8. Emphasis mine.
166. Ca.Sū.9.8.
167. "*upacārajñatā yūṣarasādikaraṇasaṃvāhanasvāpanādijñatā.*"
168. This is the very passage that Leslie and Wujastyk (1991) refer to above.
169. Ca.Sū.15.7 (first part). Translation by Dominik Wujastyk (2003, 36).
170. Ca.Sū.15.7, last part. See "The Attendant" in appendix A.
171. See Subrahmanya Ayyar 1984, 249. I would like to thank Dominik Wujastyk for bringing this epigraphical evidence to my attention.
172. Translation by Dominik Wujastyk (2003, 132–133) of Su.Kalp.1.14–18ab. See "Other Helpers" in appendix A.
173. Ca.Sū. 15.11, last part.
174. Su.Sū.34.24, Ah.Sū.1.29, and As.Sū.2.25, respectively.
175. Translation by Selby (2005, 269). See "Other Helpers" in appendix A.
176. Ibid.
177. Ca.Śā.8.37. Translation by Selby (2005, 269).
178. The medical classics suggest various methods of attempting to determine or to influence the gender of the unborn child throughout pregnancy. See Benner 2009 on the description of *saṃskāra* rites in the *Aṣṭāṅgahṛdayasaṃhitā*.
179. Kāś.Cik.18.63.
180. Su.Śā.10.25 (first part).
181. See Ca.Sū.1.120, "Other Helpers" in appendix A: "Goatherds, shepherds, cowherds, and other forest–dwellers know plants in the forest by name and form. (120) However, no one can know the best use of plants through knowing their names and forms alone. (121) One who does not even distinguish the form [of plants] but knows their application is called 'knower of truth.' However, a physician who knows plants in every respect, and (122) who knows their application, having observed on each person their effect according to place and time, is known as the best physician (123)." See also Su.Sū.36.10 (end of appendix A). "And plants can be identified by cowherds, hermits, hunters, and other forest-dwellers who eat roots."
182. See Preisendanz 2007, 629–633.
183. Preisendanz (2007, 642–652) offers a detailed comparative analysis of the differing structuring of the topic by Caraka, Suśruta and Kaśyapa.
184. Translation of Ca.Vi.8.3 by Dominik Wujastyk (2003, xxv).
185. Preisendanz 2007, 639.

186. Ca.Vi.8.68 (part) "*Jñānapūrvakaṃ hi karmaṇāṃ samārambhaṃ praśaṃsanti kuśalāḥ.*"
187. See the discussion of the quack in chapter 1.
188. See Wujastyk 2003, xxv.
189. "*Utkṛṣṭamadhyālpabuddhayas trividhāḥ śiṣyāḥ,*" Cakrapāṇidatta, Ca.Vi.8.3.
190. See Ca.Sū.4.20, and 27–28.
191. "*Vimalavipulabuddher api buddhim ākulīkuryuḥ kiṃ punar alpabuddheḥ,*" Su.Sū.4.5 (part).
192. Śār.3.13.128. Translation by Dominik Wujastyk (2003, 255).
193. Compare Suśruta's *kleśasama* in Sū.2.3.
194. In fact, Caraka copies Sū.29.7 in part of this list.
195. Kāś.Vi.2(?).5. The use of *dauṣ* is unclear here. I am treating it as the *vṛddhi* form of *duṣ*, a rare neuter form of *doṣa*, "deficiency."
196. Ca.Vi.8.5.
197. Kaśyapa then, however, begins a new passage with a change of perspective, in which the teacher addresses the student on how to behave, which correlates to some extent to Caraka's short summary of Vi.8.5., and more closely to Ca.Vi.8.13. I will look at this passage more closely in the context of the medical student's initiation.
198. Thematically, this does not belong to the preliminaries of medical study, since it describes a time when the student has already begun his studies. However, I will continue following the order in which Caraka presents his themes, in which a discussion of the preliminaries of medical study is resumed after this section.
199. Cakrapāṇidatta glosses *vacanaśakti* with *arthakīrtanasāmarthya*, "ability to express the meaning." See also Preisendanz (2007, 639–641), who paraphrases this sentence and discusses it in detail. Preisendanz also notes that the use of the second *bhūyas* does not occur in the core group of manuscripts that seem to represent the original text of the Vimānasthāna.
200. See Kane (1968–77, 2.326) on the sipping of water (*ācamana* instead of *spṛśya* in the sources he discusses) before commencing study. See also Scharfe (2002, 104), citing Oldenberg (1886, 66): "Eating water means sipping after having eased oneself." This also explains Caraka's *avaśyaka*, "necessary."
201. Literally: "going through it with words that are preceded by thought."
202. This passage has also been translated and discussed by Preisendanz (2007, 649–650).
203. "*Ātmanā cānupaṭhet paṭhataḥ śiṣyasya paścād ācāryaḥ svayaṃ paṭhet śiṣyasya sukhapaṭhanārtham,*" "'And he should repeat them by himself': After the student's reciting, the teacher should recite himself for the sake of the student's reciting easily."
204. Su.Sū.4.5.
205. Su.Sū.4.3–4.

206. As Preisendanz further notes, the topic of when study in general may not be taken up is discussed by Caraka in his chapter on good conduct (Ca.Sū.8.24). The passages in the *Suśrutasaṃhitā* and the *Kāśyapasaṃhitā* that give prescriptions on the correct times for study are Su.Sū.2.9–10 and Kāś.Vi.2.(?)7. The former reads: "One should not study on the eighth day in the dark half-month, and the two days at its end, and likewise in the bright half-month, at dawn and dusk, when there is an unseasonable roar of lightning and thunder, when there is trouble [affecting] one's own, the country, or the king, (9) on cremation grounds, in transit and during current battles, at festivals or when witnessing calamitous events, or on other days on which the sages do not study, and never when one is unclean." (10) See page 172 for the Sanskrit text. See also Preisendanz (2007, 645–646) on this passage.
207. Preisendanz (2007) refers to *Manusmṛti* 4.95–127, and *Yājñavalkyasmṛti* 1.142–151, as well as to the summaries of this topic by Kane (1968–77, 2.393–402), Mookerji (1947, 193–194) and Scharfe (2002, 2.219–220).
208. See Su.Sū.9. See Wujastyk (2003, 86–87) for a translation of this passage.
209. This passage (Ca.Vi.8.8) is headed by "Now, the method of teaching." This is somewhat confusing, since the passage immediately following the title describes the characteristics of an eligible student and does not touch on any teaching methodology. However, the heading follows the categorization set out in Ca.Vi.8.6 and comprises all of Ca.Vi.8.8–14. This will be discussed below.
210. I.e., "who promotes the true meaning." Unfortunately Cakrapāṇidatta does not supply an interpretation for what the term *arthatattvabhāvaka* might refer to. According to the findings of the Vienna project "Philosophy and Medicine in Early Classical India II," *arthatattvabhāvaka* occurs only in two of fifty-three manuscripts of the *Carakasaṃhitā* (both manuscripts from the Sarasvati Bhavan in Varanasi, nos. 108824 and 108685). In reference to Ca.Vi.8.7, the Āyurvedīya Śabdakośa explains *arthatattva* with "*viṣayasya niścitaṃ jñānaṃ siddhānto vā*," "certain knowledge or settled opinion on a subject."
211. The addition in brackets follows Cakrapāṇidatta's explanation that according to some, *anurākta* refers to study (*adhyāyanānurāga*), and according to others to the teacher (*gurāv anuraktatva*).
212. See Su.Sū.2.3, in appendix B: "A physician should initiate any brahmin, someone from the ruling classes [*kṣatriya*] or someone from the trade classes [*vaiśya*] from a good family who has youth, a good character, courage, pure habits, discipline, strength and vigor, intelligence, resolution, mindfulness, thought and perception, whose tongue, lips, and tips of teeth are thin, whose face, eyes, and nose are straight, whose mind, voice, and movements are gracious and who is equal to distress. Hence, he should not initiate one with the opposite qualities."
213. Su.Sū.2.5: "A brahmin can initiate the three (twice-born) classes, a member of the ruling classes (*kṣatriya*) the two, a member of the trade classes (*vaiśya*)

a member of the trade classes: one may even teach a member of the serving classes (*śūdra*), if he comes from a good family, without using mantras, according to some." See page 172 for the Sanskrit text of this passage. See also Scharfe 2002, 257.

214. "A student who is devoted to his preceptor, diligent and extraordinarily endowed with intelligence, mindfulness and cleverness, whose mouth, nose, and eyes are straight, and whose nails and skin are delicate and smooth (2), who leads the austere life of a student and has overcome doubt, who is intelligent, virtuous, and steadfast, who has passed six months [like this], and is possessed of modesty, [and] cleanliness and comes from a good family should be taught in the bright half of the lunar month until he has understood the meaning and the practical application of the discipline (3–4ab)." See the end of appendix B.
215. See Kāś.Vi.2(?).4, the end of appendix B: "Now for the qualities of the student: [These are] patience, skill, dexterity, suitableness, cleanliness, good birth and family, virtue, truthfulness, nonviolence, gentleness, good fortune, knowledge, discernment, steadiness, focus [*viniveśa*], cleverness, doing as told, leading the austere life of a student (i.e., celibacy etc.), humility, desisting from greed and envy. Otherwise, one with faults must be avoided."
216. Hā.1.20. See Preisendanz 2007, 632, especially note 23.
217. Kane 1968–77, 2.330.
218. Ibid.
219. Olivelle 2005, 100. See also Kane 1968–77, 2.330.
220. Olivelle 2005, 100.
221. Kane 1968–77, 2.330.
222. See Kane 1968–77, 2.327.
223. The passages Ca.Vi.8.9–14 and Su.Sū.2.4–10 are separated here into several sections for a comparison with their parallels in As.Sū.2.4 and Kāś.Vi.2(?).3. In the corresponding part of the appendix, these passages are not divided into corresponding parts, but are given as a whole. The correspondence of sequential order is picked up again in the section "The Suśrutasaṃhitā on Physicians' Professional Conduct" and is followed through to the end of the chapter.
224. See the introduction of this dissertation and Preisendanz (2007, 634–638) for an overview of the history of editions, translations, and analyses of Ca.Vi.8.
225. Preisendanz 2007.
226. Preisendanz 2007, 652.
227. Preisendanz 2007, 657: app. 3.
228. Preisendanz 2007, 660–663: app. 4.
229. The categorization of this section under the heading of "Teaching" follows Caraka's own proposed categorization. As noted, Caraka heads Vi.8.8 with "*Athādhyāpanavidhiḥ*" ("Now the rules for teaching") and ends Vi.8.14 with its corresponding "*ity adhyāpanavidhir uktaḥ*" ("Thus the rules for teaching have been stated").

230. The term *karaṇa* is only translated very loosely here. It does not correspond to the division of the day into morning, afternoon, evening, etc, that is perhaps suggested by my translation of "part of the day" but denotes a more intricate astrological division of the days of the lunar calendar. There are eleven *karaṇa*, which occupy different lengths of time at different times of the lunar month.
231. Just like *karaṇa*, the term *muhūrta* also denotes a more specific measure and moment of time. A *muhūrta* is one-thirtieth of the day, and about forty-eight minutes long.
232. Cakrapāṇidatta explains *hiraṇya* with *aghaṭitaṃ hema*, "unprocessed gold," and glosses *heman* with *ghaṭita*, "processed [gold]."
233. *Eragrostis cynosuroides Beauv.*, A sacred grass used at specific religious ceremonies.
234. Probably jasmine.
235. Kane (1968–77, 2.277) writes that a number of *nakṣatras* were considered the proper ones for initiation ceremonies. He lists *hasta, citrā, svāti, puṣya* (i.e., *tiṣya*), *dhaniṣṭhā, aśvinī* (i.e., *aśvayuj*), *mṛgaśiras, punarvasu, śravaṇa*, and *revatī* as the most commonly recommended ones, but notes that prescriptions for the time of the year varied widely, and were allocated differently according to the class of the *brahmacārin*.
236. I.e., *uttaraphālgunī*, the twelfth lunar mansion consisting of two stars, and *uttarabhādrapad(ā)*, the twenty-sixth lunar mansion, also consisting of two stars.
237. See Kane 1968–77, 2.285.
238. See Kane 1968–77, 2.278–279.
239. These are the specifications of Āpastamba Dharmasūtra (1.1.2.39–1.1.3.1–2) according to Kane (1968–77, 2.278, especially note 645). The Āśvalāyana Gṛhyasūtra gives the same instructions (see Kane 1968–77, 2.281). Other *gṛhyasūtras* prescribe white or undyed undergarments.
240. See Scharfe 2002, 107.
241. Su.Sū.2.4. prescribes *khadira* (cutch tree), *palāśa* (flame of the forest), *devadāru* (deodar), and *bilva* (Indian quince). Kāś.Vi.2(?).3. lists only *palāśa* (flame of the forest).
242. Kane (1968–77, 2.308) lists *palāśa, aśvattha, nyagrodha, plakṣa, vaikaṅkata, udumbara, bilva, candana, sarala, śāla, devadāru*, and *khadira* as prescribed types of wood for sacrifices.
243. See Kane 1968–77, 2.270.
244. Kane (1968–77, 2.285) writes: "Ap.gr.(X.5), Baud.gr.(II.5.7) and Par.gr. (II.2) prescribe a dinner to brahmanas before the ceremonies begin."
245. I.e., a prescribed rite of passage.
246. See Kane 1968–77, 2.305–306.
247. A *kiṣku* is a measure of length from the elbow to the tip of the middle finger equaling about eighteen inches. It equals a *hasta* (see Su.Sū.2.4).

248. Ca.Vi.8.11, first part.
249. *Palāśa—Butea monosperma, (Lam.) Taub.* Also called bastard teak (Griffiths 1994, 177 and Warrier et al. 1994–96, 1.314).
250. *Iṅguda—Balanites aegyptiaca?* See http://envis.frlht.org/plant_details.php?disp_id=271 and http://zipcodezoo.com/Plants/B/Balanites_aegyptiaca. It may also be *Terminalia catappa*, Indian almond. See http://envis.frlht.org/plant_details.php?disp_id=2071.
251. *Udumbara—Ficus racemosa, L.* (Sivarajan and Balachandran, 1994, 487).
252. *Madhūka—Madhuca longifolia (Koenig) Macbride* or *Bassia longifolia J. Koenig* (Warrier et al. 1994–96, 3.362).
253. Ca.Vi.8.11–12.
254. See also Scharfe (2002, 103) who gives a potted summary of the *brahmacārin*'s initiation.
255. Scharfe (2002, 259, note 39) suggests that the elaborate ritual may point to both teacher and student being envisioned as brahmins.
256. The term *tithi* describes a lunar day, i.e., a day of thirty in the lunar month.
257. Ḍalhaṇa explains that the auspiciousness of date and time should be ascertained by astrologers.
258. A *hasta* is a measure of length from the elbow to the tip of the middle finger equaling about eighteen inches.
259. Ḍalhaṇa writes *ullikhya ūrdhvamukhīṃ lekhāṃ kṛtvā.*
260. *abhyukṣya jalena siktvā*, according to Ḍalhaṇa.
261. Or "Placing [a symbol of] the Absolute to the right"? The meaning of this is not clear to me, and it seems that it was also not clear to Suśruta's commentator Ḍalhaṇa, who omits the words "*brahmāṇaṃ sthāpayitvā*" altogether, although he gives a detailed word-to-word commentary on this passage otherwise.
262. *Khadira—Acacia catechu.* See http://envis.frlht.org/plant_details.php?disp_id=22 and http://zipcodezoo.com/Plants/A/Acacia_catechu/. See also Warrier et al. 1994–96, 1.19.
263. *Devadāru—Cedrus deodara.* See http://envis.frlht.org/plant_details.php?disp_id=485 and Warrier et al. 1994–96, 2.41.
264. *Bilva—Aegle marmelos.* See http://envis.frlht.org/plant_details.php?disp_id=63. According to Warrier et al. (1994–96, 1.62), the English name is bael tree or holy fruit tree.
265. *Nyagrodha—Ficus bengalensis.* See http://envis.frlht.org/plant_details.php?disp_id=969.
266. *Aśvattha—Ficus religiosa.* See http://envis.frlht.org/plant_details.php?disp_id=987.
267. *Upanayanīyaṃ tu brāhmaṇaṃ* at the beginning of this *sūtra.*
268. *Prāk brāhmaṇagrahaṇaṃ varṇeṣu madhye tasya śreṣṭhatvāt.*
269. See Kane's summaries of fire rituals, in which most of the terminology used by Kaśyapa (*agnipraṇayana, parisamūhana, paryukṣaṇa, paristaraṇa [āstaraṇa],*

ājyotpavana, āghāra) are found. See Kane 1968–77, 2.207–211, esp. 210–211, and also Gonda 1980, 167.

270. I.e., *uttaraphālgunī*, the twelfth lunar mansion consisting of two stars, and *uttarabhādrapad(ā)*, the twenty-sixth lunar mansion, also consisting of two stars.
271. According to MW., the measure of a cow hide (*gocarmamātra*) can mean a very large surface area, but may have originally denoted "a piece of land large enough to be encompassed by straps of leather from a cow's hide." The latter meaning seems to fit the context of a ceremonial platform better than the former. See also Ḍalhaṇa's commentary on Su.Sū.2.4, in which he discusses the uses of *gocarmamātra* as a measure either denoting the grounds on which the ceremonial platform is built or the platform itself. In the latter case, he equates *gocarmamātra* with the measure that Suśruta gives for the platform: namely *caturhasta*.
272. The oblations specified are the two *āghāra* oblations, which are offerings of clarified butter to Prajāpati and to Indra (see Kane 1968–77, 2.211, note 489), and the *ājya* (clarified butter) oblations to Agni and to Soma (see Kane 1968–77, 2.207, note 283).
273. According to MW. (giving Ṛgveda 4.39.6 as a reference), *dadhikrāvan*, or *dadhikrā*, is the name of a divine horse, a personification of the morning sun.
274. Kāś.Vi 2(?).6: "Now the instruction for the student: O! You should be placid, friendly, virtuous, have mastered your senses, and study when summoned. You should tell [me] everything, sympathize [with me], know the right place and time and be resolute. You should turn away from anger, avarice, arrogance, envy, derision, animosity, alcohol, meat, and women. You should study as one of whom [only] obedience to his preceptor remains. If you have not received permission [to leave], and have not worshiped [your] preceptor, and if you have incomplete knowledge, you must not be allowed to roam around [practicing medicine]."
275. Menon and Haberman (1970) note that their division of the text partly follows "appropriate titles" and partly is "arbitrarily divided." See also the brief discussion by Preisendanz (2007, 637–638) on Haberman and Menon's article.
276. This division comprises eight subdivisions.
277. Preisendanz (2007, 638) also makes note of further classifications of this passage by Athavale and Athavale (2003: 14–17) into four sections (which does not reflect the structure of the text, but its contents), and by Ramachandra Rao (1985: 121–122), who "isolates nineteen points of instruction in medical ethics in the master's speech."
278. Ca.Vi.8.13, first part.
279. Olivelle 1999, 10.
280. See Olivelle 1999, 81.
281. See Olivelle 2005, 37.

282. Olivelle 1999, 137.
283. Unfortunately, we also learn nothing more from Cakrapāṇidatta's commentary, which does not discuss this passage in detail.
284. Su.Sū.2.6.
285. Some of Suśruta's requirements are, however, mentioned by Caraka in his instructions on the student's behavior as a practitioner.
286. See Kane (1968–77, 2.370–373) for an overview of *vratas* observed as part of studentship.
287. Or, in accordance with my translation of *brahmacārin* in Ca.Vi.8.13: "the austere life of a student." However, *brahmacārya* as an umbrella term would include rules about observances and salutations, so that its narrower translation "celibacy" seems more appropriate to me here.
288. See, for example, Kane (1968–77, 2.335–343) on the intricate rules on correct salutation for the *brahmacārin*.
289. See Āpastamba Dharmasūtra 1.4.22–29 (Olivelle, 1999, 12), Gautama Dharmasūtra 2.22 (Olivelle, 1999, 81), Baudhāyana Dharmasūtra 1.3.22 (Olivelle, 1999, 136). See also Scharfe (2002, 233).
290. See, for example, *Gautama Dharmasūtra* 2.24., *Manusmṛti* 2.119, and *Viṣṇusmṛti* 28.24, according to Scharfe (2002, 235).
291. See Scharfe (2002, 235), paraphrasing *Manusmṛti* 2.199 and *Viṣṇusmṛti* 28.25.
292. The other authors give corresponding advice (which will be discussed as well), but not in the context of the initiation speech. In the case of the *Suśrutasaṃhitā*, there is some ambiguity in this regard. The teacher's vow in Su.Sū.2.7, which seems to conclude his speech at the initiation ceremony, is followed by a passage on whom to treat and whom not to treat, and one on the right times for study. These could be understood as part of the teacher's speech, but since there is a change in address from the teacher addressing the student in the second person in the preceding passage (Su.Sū.2.6–7) to prescriptions in the third person, I do not interpret these sections (i.e., Su.Sū.8–10) as part of the initiation speech.
293. Cakrapāṇidatta explains *pravicaritavyam* with *cikitsārthaṃ vyavahartavyam*, "it is to be roamed for the sake of medical practice."
294. Ca.Vi.8.13–14.
295. The title Preisendanz (2007, 660–662) has given to this section, "Student's Behaviour as a Practitioner (Already during the Period of Apprenticeship?)," reflects this ambiguity.
296. See, for example, the famous *Metta Sutta* of the Pāli Canon. In this discourse on loving kindness, prayers for the happiness of all beings play a central role. See Suttapiṭaka, Khuddakanikāya, Suttanipāta 1.8., for example in Norman 1992, 16-17. See also my notes on Ca.Sū.9.26 regarding the Buddhist *brahmavihāra*.
297. See chapter 1.
298. Su.Sū.2.8.

299. See note 292.
300. As.Sū.2.18–19. All of these passages are discussed in chapter 1.
301. On messengers, see Ca.Ind.12.9–24, and chapter 4.
302. This dictum is reiterated in Ca.Ind.12.62–64. This is discussed in more detail in chapter 6.
303. Ca.Sū.8.32. *Nṛlokam āpūrayate yaśasā sādhusaṃmataḥ | dharmārthāveti bhūtānāṃ bandhutām upagacchati* (32).
304. Ca.Sū.8.25 (part). *Na guhyaṃ vivṛṇuyāt na kañcid avajānīyāt nāhaṃmānī syān nādakṣo nādakṣiṇo nāsūyakaḥ*, "One should not disclose a secret, one should not treat anyone with contempt, one should not be conceited, or unskilled, or incompetent, or envious."
305. Ca.Sū.8.18 (part). *Devagobrāhmaṇaguruvṛddhasiddhācāryān arcayet.*
306. Su.Sū.2.7.
307. Translation by Dominik Wujastyk (2003, 88, 90).
308. See Su.Cik.24.89.
309. Kāś.Vi.2.(?)9 concerns debate with colleagues, which also forms part of physicians' etiquette. This is discussed separately.
310. It is not clear to me what the "other" (*para*) is in Kaśyapa's *parādhīna*, i.e., whether this refers to another medicine, or to another person on whom the physician must not depend in making his medicine.
311. The meaning of *upanayavad* is not entirely clear here. *Upanaya* is a term from the Nyāya system of logic. The Nyāya school of philosophical speculation is one of the six orthodox schools of Hindu philosophy. According to this system, there are four sources of knowledge (*pramāṇa*): perception, inference, comparison, and testimony. The methodology of inference (*anumāna*) involves a combination of induction and deduction by moving from particular to particular via generality. It has five steps, one of which is *upanaya*, which has been translated as "summarizing statement" ("zusammenfassende Bemerkung") by Prets and Prandstetter (1991–, 2.36–39) in the context of Nyāyasūtra 1.1.38. More precisely, *upanaya* denotes the defining of example and the object of the hypothesis, or their respective qualities as analogous. This is also how it is used in the *Carakasaṃhitā* (Vi.8.27). Caraka's example runs as follows: Hypothesis: The Puruṣa is eternal. Reason: Because it has not been produced. Example: Like the ether (which is eternal). Statement of analogy (*upanaya*): Just as the ether has not been produced and is eternal, the Puruṣa has not been produced and is eternal. Conclusion: The Puruṣa is eternal. The *upanayavad* of Kaśyapa's text then may refer to this step in the methodology of inference, i.e., proposing an analogy that shows something to be as asserted. More simply, it may refer to providing examples and analogies to prove one's point.
312. However, Ca.Vi.8.15, i.e., the passage that immediately follows the teacher's speech, gives guidelines on how to conduct debate with colleagues. This is paralleled by a much shorter passage in Kāś.Vi.2(?).9.

313. I.e., a treatise on practical life and political government. It is not certain whether this alludes to the work attributed to Kauṭilya or to some other work.
314. The text gives *hreṣaṇīyāṃ* here, which translates as "to be whinnied," i.e., the gerundive of the root *hreṣ*, "to neigh" or "to whinny." This meaning obviously does not fit the context, and I think it unlikely that "whinnying" stands in lieu of "laughing" here, i.e., "to be laughed [about]," which would fit better. I rather assume that *hreṣaṇīyāṃ* is a false reading. I suggest the alternative reading *hrepayanīyāṃ*, "shaming" or "embarrassing," the adjective used without gerundive character.
315. As.Sū.2.7–19.
316. According to Scharfe (2002, 87), "the custom and the term (of *upanayana*) can be traced from early Vedic texts to modern times . . . Its roots can even be traced to still earlier times, because the Avesta and the Zoroastrian tradition have a similar custom." See also Kane (1968–77, 2.268 and 271–272) on the oldest sources of the terms and concepts of *brahmacarya* and *upanayana*.
317. A *brahmacārin*'s initiation is seen as his second birth (the first being his physical birth), and he is therefore henceforth called a "twice-born" (*dvija*). See Kane 1968–77, 2.189.
318. See,for example, Ca.Sū.8.20, 21, and 23, Ca.Sū.15.9, Ca.Nid.7.14, Ca.Vi.8.14, Ca.Śa.8.13, Su.Sū.2.8, Su.Sū.3.50, Su.Sū.32.4, Su.Utt.60.9 to name just a few instances where *dvijas* are mentioned.
319. Scharfe refers to BauDhS 1.2,6 and VasDhS 2.6 and Manu. 2.172.
320. See Manu. 3.152, 3.180, and 3.169–179, respectively (Olivelle 2005, 116–117).
321. Jolly (1994 [1951], 27) points to counterexamples in Buddhist sources, where the physician Jīvaka Komārabaccha, a contemporary of the Buddha, is described as highly respected for his skills as a physician. On Jīvaka see also Zysk 2000, 52–61. From Zysk's summary of the Jīvaka legend in the Pāli Canon, we can see that physicians may have generally had a positive image. There is for, example, mention of a "world-famous" physician in Taxila, with whom Jīvaka studied for seven years. However, since the topic of the medical student's initiation has more in common with brahmanic sources than with Buddhist ones, it makes more sense to compare the medical authors' views with brahmanic sources here.
322. On the idea that the origins of Ayurveda lie outside brahmanic culture, going back to ascetic intellectuals, see Zysk (2000) and Chattopadhyaya (1977). Zysk (2000, 4) writes that "the traditional account of Indian medicine is merely the result of a later Hinduization process applied to a fundamentally heterodox body of knowledge to render it orthodox." The fact that some brahmins did become physicians is, for example, attested by the existence of the *Aṣṭavaidyas*, Keralan brahmin families whose male members traditionally practice Ayurveda.
323. Wujastyk adds "brahmin" in brackets here, since *dvija* often denotes persons of the brahmin class. However, while it is certainly possible that the physician in

question may have been brahmin, the interpretation of "twice-born" as brahmin does not make sense here, since it is in the very next sentence defined differently: a physician becomes a twice-born by completing his studies.

324. Translation by Dominik Wujastyk (1993, 762) of Ca.Cik.1.51–53 (see appendix E for the Sanskrit text).
325. Trikamji chooses the readings *dvijātiḥ* (twice-born) in Cik.1.51, *dvitīyā* (second) in 52, and *dvijaḥ* (twice-born) in 53, but notes that there are alternate readings with *trijātiḥ* (thrice-born) in 51, *tṛtīyā* (third) in 52, and *trijaḥ* (thrice-born) in 53. The latter is the reading favored by Sharma in his edition and translation. Trikamji's rendering of Cakrapāṇidatta's commentary reads "twice-born" etc.
326. See Ca.Vi.8.8.
327. See Su.Sū.2.3–5.
328. Most notably by Menon and Haberman (1970). See also Jonsen (2000, 30).
329. See Benner 2005b, 188. See also Preisendanz 2007, 637–638.
330. "Und so wissen wir denn genau, dass der Ehevertrag durch a) das Sprechen der (Vertrags)worte, b) das Ausgiessen von Wasser, c) das Reichen der rechten Hand, d) die rechtswendige Umrundung eines Feuers, e) das Opfern in dieses und f) das gemeinsame Schreiten von 7 Schritten geschlossen wurde" (Oberlies, 2002, 72). These elements are described in the context of marriages, but Oberlies argues that the marriage ceremony may serve as a blueprint for contracts in general.
331. See Oberlies 2002, 72. Also see Hopkins 1932, 324, on the fire as witness.
332. On the pouring of water on hands see Oberlies (2002, 77), and on the use of water in regard to oaths see Hopkins (1932, 324–326).
333. Compare Ah.Sū.2.31–31 and Su.Cik.24.89–90.
334. See Vāgbhaṭa's chapter on daily regimen (*dinacaryā*), and particularly As.Sū.3.41–42.
335. See Manu. 4.35–36 (Olivelle, 2005, 126) and Baudhāyana Dharmasūtra 5.1–7 (Olivelle, 1999, 139).
336. See Oldenberg 1886, 91.
337. See Olivelle 2005, 131.
338. Olivelle 2005, 131.
339. See Su.Sū.4.6–7.
340. See Ca.Vi.8.6.
341. Suśruta presents debate with colleagues as a requirement for entering the profession (see Su.Sū.10.3), but he does not discuss this any further.
342. Cakrapāṇidatta gives *spardhā*–"competition" or "rivalry"—for *saṃharṣa* (Trikamji Acarya, 1992a, 265), which I would otherwise translate as "joy." However, the word *saṃharṣa* appears again later in juxtaposition with *vijigīṣu*, "wishing to win," which rather corroborates the meaning of "competition" than that of "joy." Karin Preisendanz has noted that the critical edition of Ca.Vi.8

prepared in Vienna reads *saṃgharṣa*, "rivalry" (personal communication by email, July 9, 2009).

343. Cakrapāṇidatta glosses *bhūyo 'dhyavasāyam* with *dṛḍhaniścayam*—"firm conviction."
344. See note 342 on *saṃharṣa*.
345. See Ca.Vi.8.15–66.
346. See Wujastyk (2007–8) and Preisendanz (2009) for summaries of Caraka's description of debate methodology.
347. Kaśyapa describes debate among colleagues in a similar, though much shorter passage in Vi.2(?).9.
348. Wujastyk in preparation.
349. Ca.Vi.8.67, first part.
350. Ca.Vi.8.67.
351. "They do not wish to question, nor to be questioned, and shrink from questions as from death. And no one is known as their teacher, pupil, co-student, or disputant." See the discussion of the quack in chapter 1.
352. See Su.Sū.34.19cd–21ab.
353. See Ca.Sū.1.
354. The term used for "kindness" is *maitrī*; see Ca.Sū.1.30. The terms used for "compassion" are *anukrośa*, see Ca.Sū.1.7 and Ca.Sū.1.35; *anukampā*, see Ca.Sū.1.30; and *kāruṇya*, see Ca.Cik.1.4.4. The *Suśrutasaṃhitā* gives a similar account to Caraka's in Sūtrasthāna 1. It does not use any term denoting "compassion," but it is clear from its description that compassion and the wish for the welfare of humankind are at the core of the sages' quest for medical knowledge. See particularly Su.Sū.1.4. A similar version of the origins of Ayurveda also occurs at the beginning of the *Bhāvaprakāśa*. All of these are discussed in Zysk 1999.
355. See Ca.Sū.8.29, Ah.Sū.2.27, and Ah.Sū.2.46. It is notable that there are no comparable statements in the *Suśrutasaṃhitā*.
356. I.e., those who are healthy. As noted in chapter 1, Cakrapāṇidatta suggests a rather different meaning for *prakṛtistha*: "approaching death."
357. Ca.Sū.9.26. This is part of Caraka's four-pillar definition. As.Utt.50.196 paraphrases Caraka's passage.
358. Ah.Śā.5.131.
359. See also Meulenbeld 1999–2002, IA:609 and IB:686.
360. See Ca.Ind.1–4.
361. Ca.Ind.4.
362. See Ca.Ind.5–10.
363. See Ca.Ind.12.
364. See Ca.Ind.5.20, 5.47, 6.13, 6.14, 7.15, 7.19, 7.25, 8.15, 9.9, 9.13, 9.14, 11.22, 12.9, 12.11, 12.14, 12.17, 12.21, 12.31, and 12.64. The other authors give similar injunctions to abandon a patient with an incurable disease or wound: See, for

example, Su.Sū.28.13–15 and 21, 31.14 and 22, 33.11. Also see Ah.Śā.5.1–3, 40, 95, 113–116, 121–122. The admonition to abandon a patient from afar occurs in Ca.Ind.7.15 and 9.14.

365. See, for example, Ca.Ind.8.4–7 (patient will die within either three or six days) Ca.Ind.9.22 (patient will die within three fortnights), Ca.Ind.10.3–20 (patient will die soon and suddenly), Ca.Ind.11.6 (patient will die within a year), Ca.Ind.11.8 (patient will die within half a year), Ca.Ind.11.12 (patient will die within a month), and Ca.Ind.12.5 (the patient will die within a fortnight).
366. See, for example, Ca.Sū.1.62, also Ca.Sū.10.7–8, and Su.Sū.10.6 and Su.Sū.28.21.
367. See Ca.Sū.10.9.
368. See Ca.Sū.10.17–18, as well as Ah.Sū.1.32, and As.Sū.2.30.
369. See Su.Sū.23.9–11.
370. See Su.Sū.10.6.
371. See note 73.
372. As.Śā.7.29–31. Meulenbeld (1999–2002, IA:607) makes note of this passage in a discussion on diseases classified as curable, incurable, or *yāpya*.
373. Ah.Śā.5.130. For parallel passages see Su.Sū.31.31–32, Ca.Ind.11.25–27, and Bhāv.Pūrv.6.86–87.
374. Ca.Sū.10.8.
375. *Tasminn upekṣā kartavyā; na tatra bheṣajadānādi kartavyaṃ, yaśohānyādibhayāt.*
376. Ca.Vi.3.45. See the discussion of patients to reject in chapter 1.
377. Su.Sū.28.7.
378. See Meulenbeld 1999–2002, IB:686, note 197.
379. See K.A.4.1.56–57 (Kangle, 1972, 258).
380. These punishments are listed in K.A. 3.19.12–14.
381. Su.Sū.10.3. See "The *Suśrutasaṃhitā* on Physicians' Professional Conduct" in chapter 2.
382. See, for example, Su.Cik.15.3, in which Suśruta says that in the case of having to remove a badly positioned fetus from the womb, a physician must first ask the king for permission. There are also a number of passages in which a disease is first declared to be incurable before the physician embarks on treatment. The key word here is *pratyākhyāya*, "having rejected," which seems to be used in the sense of "having proclaimed [it] rejectable," i.e., pointing out that the disease is incurable. See also Su.Sū.28.21, Su.Cik.21.18 and 22.81, Ca.Si.9.73, and Ah.Śa.2.6.
383. Ca.Cik.13.175–178.
384. Ca.Cik.23 deals with snakes, their poisons and the treatments against snake bite poisoning.
385. The epigraph is from Benjamin Jowett's translation, at http://classics.mit.edu/Plato/republic.2.i.html (Web site consulted December 2008).

386. Ah.Śā.6.72–73ab. See the discussion of the patient demographic in chapter 1.
387. See the discussion of the patient demographic and patients to reject in chapter 1, regarding Ca.Vi.3.45, that poor people should not be treated and Cakrapāṇidatta's commentary that medical treatment cannot be done since poor people lack the equipment for it. Also see Su.Sū.10.8, that poor persons are difficult to treat, and Ḍalhaṇa's explanation that this is so because they cannot afford medicines. Further, see Ca.Si.2.5, warning not to treat patients who lack equipment, and As.Sū.2.18cd–19.
388. Wujastyk 1993, 762. See the discussion of the quack in chapter 1.
389. As.Utt.50.192: "No other gift excels the gift of life. Therefore, [the physician] should treat the poor and ascetics with his very own resources."
390. See the discussion of the patient demographic in chapter 1.
391. See Su.Sū.34.19cd–21ab, Ca.Sū.29.7, and Ca.Vi.8.86.
392. Siegel (1985, 182) summarizes this passage. Also see Basham 1998 [1976], 23–24.
393. Cakrapāṇidatta explains *vidvadgrahaṇayaśaḥ* with *vidvadupādeyatājanyaṃ yaśa[s]*, "renown arising from the acceptance by the wise."
394. There is a very similar passage in the *Kāśyapasaṃhitā* (Vi.2(?).10, middle part), which includes *śūdras* among those who are to practice medicine: "By whom should it be studied?" Āyurveda should be studied by brahmins, by those of the governing classes [*kṣatriya*], by those of the trade classes [*vaiśya*] and by those of the serving classes [*śūdra*]. To this end: By brahmins for the sake of thorough knowledge, for their own merit, and in order to assist living beings, by those of the governing classes to protect their subjects, by those of the trade classes for a living, by the rest as service, and by all for the sake of virtue." Compare also *Manusmṛti* 1.87–91 on the proper occupations of the social classes: "For the protection of this whole creation, that One of dazzling brilliance assigned separate activities for those born from the mouth, arms, thighs, and feet. To Brahmins, he assigned reciting and teaching the Veda, offering and officiating at sacrifices, and receiving and giving gifts. To the Kṣatriya, he allotted protecting the subjects, giving gifts, offering sacrifices, reciting the Veda, and avoiding attachment to sensory objects; and to the Vaiśya, looking after animals, giving gifts, offering sacrifices, reciting the Veda, trade, moneylending and agriculture. A single activity did the Lord allot to the Śūdra, however: the ungrudging service of those very social classes" (Olivelle, 2005, 91).
395. Zysk 2000, 45.
396. Kangle 1972, 56: Ṛtvigācāryapurohitaśrotriyebhyo brahmadeyāny adaṇḍa-karāṇy abhirūpadāyādakāni prayacchet—adhyakṣasaṃkhyāyakādibhyo gopasthānikānīkasthacikitsakāśvadamakajaṅghākārikebhyaś ca vikrayādhāna-varjāni.
397. Kangle 1972, 295.

398. I have already mentioned this inscription in the context of nursing staff. See the discussion of the attendant and other helpers in chapter 1.
399. Subrahmanya Ayyar (1984, 249).
400. That the physician works alone is not evident from the passage quoted from the *Arthaśāstra* above. However, in the few instances in which the physician is mentioned in the *Arthaśāstra*, there is no mention of a hospital setting for his work.
401. "A person who has been treated, but does not recompense the physician, still owes him, whether agreed to or not" (Ca.Cik.1.55).
402. Bhāv.Pūrv.6.35.
403. Ca.Cik.1.59. The same verse also occurs in As.Utt.50.190.
404. See Bhāv.Pūrv.6.34: "Medicine should not be practiced as a trade out of greed. However, one may wish to obtain money for a livelihood from lords and wealthy persons."
405. See Bhāv.Pūrv.6.37 and 89.
406. See Ca.Sū.5.104: "One should take up such means of livelihood as are not incompatible with virtue. That way, one attains peace and study as well as happiness." Caraka gives examples of such means of livelihood in Sū.11.5, where he states that "one should learn about and begin to practice agriculture, animal husbandry, trade, service to the king, etc., and indeed any other occupations that are approved by the good and that cause an increase in livelihood. This way, a person lives a long life without dishonor."
407. There is a parallel passage in As.Sū.3.38cd–40ab.
408. See, for example, Su.Sū.10.8 and 25.45, Ca.Ind.12.90 and Ca.Ni.8.37.
409. Trikamji reads *cārthakāmārtham*, "for the sake of wealth and pleasure," but notes the alternate reading of *nārthakāmārtham*, "*not* for the sake of wealth and pleasure," which is favored by Sharma.
410. Ca.Cik.1.56–58.
411. Ca.Cik.1.60–62. Translation by Dominik Wujastyk 1993, 762.
412. Ca.Sū.9.26.
413. Bhāv.Pūrv.6.32. As.Utt.50.194 reads nearly the same: "In some cases it is virtue, in others friendship, or wealth, fame or the practice of medical treatment; thus medicine is never without reward."
414. Beauchamp and Childress 2001, 12.
415. For the sake of brevity, I will refer to the doctor as "he."
416. Su.Sū.25.43–44. This passage is oddly placed within a chapter on the eight types of surgical operations, where it does not at all fit in with the general context. For a similar statement about the doctor–patient relationship see As.Utt.50.189: "A diligent physician should protect all patients who are suffering as he would his own children, keeping in mind knowledge and virtue."
417. Ca.Sū.8.19.

418. Word searches for the same keywords were also conducted in the *Mādhava-nidāna*, the *Bhāvaprakāśa*, and the *Śārṅgadharasaṃhitā* but did not bring up any relevant results.
419. For an excellent complete translation of this chapter see Wujastyk (2003, 38–50).
420. The translation of *kṛtayuga* as "Golden Age" is not literal but follows the common modern usage of the concept of the Golden Age, i.e., a utopian period of peace, prosperity and happiness in the beginnings of humanity. Similarly, *tretāyuga* is translated as "Silver Age," i.e., a period regarded as notable but inferior to the Golden Age.
421. I.e., the five elements (*mahābhūta*) ether, air, fire, water, and earth.
422. The concepts of savor, potency, postdigestive savor, and specific action (*rasa, vīrya, vipāka,* and *prabhāva*) are used to explain the effects of drugs. Caraka defines these concepts in Sūtrasthāna 26. See also Meulenbeld (1987) for a discussion of their meanings.
423. Sāṃkhya is one of the six orthodox schools of classical Indian philosophy.
424. On the differences between Sāṃkhya cosmology and understanding of the *guṇas* and that of the ayurvedic authors see Scharfe (1999, esp. 622–623) and Müller (1934).
425. Cakrapāṇidatta glosses *daiva*, "divine," with *adṛṣṭa*, "invisible," "not experienced," or "that which is beyond the reach of observation or consciousness," and explains that such remedies would include the use of powerful auspicious amulets or charms, etc.
426. See by contrast Benner (2005a) on Ah.Sū.11.2 on the positive interpretation of the *doṣas* as an essential part of the body. See also Scharfe (1999) for an overview of the differences and similarities regarding the understanding of the concept of the *doṣas* in the medical classics and other Indian literature.
427. See also Ca.Vi.6.5 and Ca.Śā.1.142 for similar statements. These are discussed at some length by Scharfe (1999, 622–623).
428. This passage is quoted nearly verbatim in Ah.Sū.4.36, merely exchanging *nara*, "a man," for *nityam*, "always." A similar passage in the chapter on "daily regimen" (*dinācārya*) in As.Sū.3.82–86a omits any mention of truthfulness, though it does not seem to abbreviate otherwise, but rather to extend explanations of a good person's behavior.
429. Cakrapāṇidatta comments *sahasā ātmaśaktim anālocyam kriyata iti sāhasaṃ, tat tu gajābhimukhadhāvanādi*, "Recklessness is acting in an unpremeditated manner without having considered one's own strength, like running towards an elephant etc."
430. See Su.Sū.2.6 in the discussion of the medical student's behavior toward his teacher in chapter 2.
431. Part of Ca.Vi.8.13. See "The Teacher's Speech and the Student's Vow" in chapter 2.

432. Ibid.
433. Part of Ca.Vi.8.13.
434. Though note, for example, the list of forbidden foods and the chapter on eating meat in Manu's Dharmaśāstra, a major work on religious law roughly dated to between the last two centuries BCE and the first two centuries CE. Here, Manu states: "He may eat meat when it is sacrificially consecrated, at the behest of Brahmins, when he is ritually commissioned according to rule, and when his life is at risk"(Olivelle, 2005, 139). The last part of this statement is particularly important for the medicinal use of meat.
435. The use of meat does, however, become an issue for the later commentators, such as Cakrapāṇidatta. See Zimmermann (1999 [1987], 192–193) and Wujastyk (2004b) for Cakrapāṇidatta's discussion of the tension between the use of meat and the ethical goal of nonviolence. It is, however, only in the *Kalyāṇakāraka*, a Jain medical work by Ugrāditya dated to c. the ninth century (Meulenbeld, 1999–2002, IIA, 155), that vegetarianism becomes the central focus of ethical argument. Here, animal products that can only be obtained through killing or harming an animal are replaced by vegetable or mineral substances, or by other animal products such as hair, nails, excrement, etc.
436. Read *vesavāra*, "particular condiment or kind of seasoning," for *veśavāra*.
437. On the changing customs regarding the eating of beef by Hindus see K.T. Achaya 1998; 16–18. On the use of beef in medicine and the implications of its use for the status of physicians in ancient India, see D. Chattopadhyaya 1977, 380–387.
438. *Vyāghrādīnām ity arthaḥ. viśuddhamanasaḥ śokakrodhādy anabhibhūtamanasa ity arthaḥ; jejjaṭas tu vyāghrādīnām māṃsāni chadmopahitāni, evaṃ viśuddhamanasa iti vyākhyānayati.*
439. This quotation is also interesting for the reason that it represents a section of Jejjaṭa's commentarial work that is otherwise not available to us at present. It is not clear whether Ḍalhaṇa's quotation of Jejjaṭa stems from the latter's commentary on Caraka, or the one on Suśruta. According to K. Zysk (personal communication by email, Nov. 14, 2006), we don't have the manuscript of Jejjaṭa's commentary on Ca.Cik.8.149–157. Meulenbeld in IA, 385, writes: "Jejjaṭa commented on both *Caraka*– and *Suśrutasaṃhitā*. His commentary on the latter treatise has partly been preserved, but its title is unknown." And in note 360 of IB, 507, Meulenbeld adds: "A single MS, containing part of the commentary on the Uttaratantra, is known (NCC VII, 317; STMI 89)."
440. Patrick Olivelle, in his translation of Manu's Dharmaśāstra, notes that "Dharma literature makes a clear distinction between *abhakṣya*, foods forbidden because of their very nature, and *abhojya*, foods that have become unfit for a variety of reasons" (Olivelle, 2005, 278, note 5.5).
441. Manu's list of forbidden foods is found in chapter 5. It includes carnivorous birds (5.11), animals that wander alone (5.17), and animals with five nails

(*pañcanākha*, 5.17–18). Interestingly the rhinoceros, despite being categorized as having five nails and wandering alone, may be eaten. The camel is specifically mentioned as a forbidden food (see Olivelle 2005, 138–139). Zimmermann (1999, 243, note 45), referring to Bhāgavata Purāṇa III, 10, 20–24, lists the *pañcanākha* animals as follows: dog, jackal, wolf, tiger, cat, hare, porcupine, lion, monkey, elephant, tortoise, lizard, and *makara* (a kind of sea monster). Further, Manu notes in chapter 11, 157, that "The hot-arduous penance is the purification for eating the meat of carnivorous animals, pigs, camels, cocks, humans, crows or donkeys," thus firmly placing carnivores into the list of forbidden foods (Olivelle, 2005, 223).

442. This, incidentally, may be what Jejjaṭa (via Ḍalhaṇa) on Su.Ci.1.82bc–83ab is hinting at when he comments that the mind remains pure because the meats are given under disguise.

443. Commenting on another passage, Cakrapāṇidatta discusses the question whether the physician commits an act of cruelty by recommending meat. First, Cakrapāṇidatta argues that "the masters of ayurveda do not actually recommend meat: they merely say that meat can be good for you in certain circumstances" (Wujastyk, 2004b, 836). Second, he states that the responsibility for eating meat lies with the eater, not with the doctor who recommends it (Wujastyk, 2004b, 836). However, Cakrapāṇidatta's general statements about the use of meat do not include a discussion about food categorization in a religious sense and also do not answer the question about liability in the case of a physician giving a patient something that the latter would not accept if he knew what it was.

444. Translation by Wujastyk 2004b, 836 of Cakrapāṇidatta *on* Ca.Sū.8.29, *na hy āyurvedavidhayo dharmasādhanam evopadiśanti, kiṃ tarhy ārogyasādhanaṃ.*

445. See, for example, Benner 2009 on brahmanic fertility rituals in the *Aṣṭāṅgahṛdayasaṃhitā*. Zysk (2000) writes comprehensively about the use of brahmanic material in the medical texts, as does Chattopadhyaya (1977).

446. Cakrapāṇidatta *on* Ca.Sū.8.19: *nānṛtaṃ brūyād ity asya rājayakṣmaṇi 'kākāṃs tittiriśabdena' ityādy ayathābhāṣaṇopadeśena virodho na vācyaḥ, yataḥ parāpakāraphalam asatyabhāṣaṇam anṛtavyāhāradoṣeṇa spṛśyate, na tu parasya jīvanārtham anyathābhāṣaṇam.* See also Zimmermann's translation, it cannot be said that there is any contradiction[,] for false speech is only affected by the vice of lying when its effect is to harm others, and is in this case it is in order to save another's life that one does not speak the truth." (Zimmermann, 1999 [1987], 178).

447. This plant is a climber with pods that are covered with irritant bristles. See http://envis.frlht.org/plant_details.php?disp_id=1471.

448. Cakrapāṇidatta glosses *siṃha* with *vyāghra*, thus interpreting it as as a tiger rather than as the nonnative lion.

449. Cakrapāṇidatta specifies that "outside" means outside the village.

450. Ca.Cik.9.79–84. This section is also described and discussed by Smith (2006, 538). Smith elsewhere (2006, 477) makes note of Caraka's categorization of madness by accountable pathological factors and madness by unaccountable invasive entities, the latter being the focus of Smith's study.
451. Zimmermann points this out in his discussion of the carnivore's meats that are given under disguise by the physician in Ca.Cik.8.149–157: "Fantastical prescriptions, I admit, if only because they presuppose a whole economic infrastructure capable of producing on demand lions, bears, hyenas, tigers, and other game—in short, a royal existence!" (Zimmermann 1999 [1987], 176).
452. The same passage appears in Mādh. 20.14–15.
453. Ca.Vi.8.13.
454. The latter topic is briefly explored in the discussion of veracity in the doctor–patient relationship in chapter 6.
455. Zimmermann 1999 [1987], 181.
456. Ibid.
457. See also Olivelle (2005, 139) on a passage in *Manusmṛti* in which exceptions to the rule of vegetarianism are listed. On this, see also the discussion of veracity in the doctor–patient relationship in chapter 6 and Wujastyk 2004b.
458. That is, other than the commentator Cakrapāṇidatta's discussion on the topic of whether the use of meat in medicine does not contradict the ideal of friendship to all beings (Ca.Cik.8.149–157), which I discuss in detail in chapter 6.
459. See, for example, Ca.Vi.3.24, which cites violence, or the infliction of injury (*abhighāta*) as one of the reasons and symptoms of worsening conditions in the world. See also Ca.Sū.7.29 (on restraining urges of violence), As.Sū.2.18–19, Bhāv.Pūrv.6.41, Ca.Vi.3.45, Ca.Si.2.4, and Ah.Sū.1.34–35ab (on a physician's avoidance of violent persons).
460. See Ca.Sū.29.7 (which says that a physician who entertains friendly thoughts toward all beings belongs to the category of "saver of life"), Kāś.Vi.2(?).4 (which states that a medical student should be gentle and nonviolent), Kāś.Sū.26.4 (which requires a physician to have friendly relations with all beings), and As.Sū.2.7 (which includes friendliness among the requirements of professional conduct).
461. One could, however, argue that Suśruta's definition in Sū.34.21–22 of the patient as someone who is resolute implies that patients' fears were taken into account by physicians.
462. See the discussion of veracity in the doctor–patient relationship in chapter 6 on this topic.
463. See Lipner 1989, 53–57.
464. See Ca.Sū.8.19.
465. On this, see Lipner 1989, 49–50. This seems to refer to the fetus's position in the womb rather than to any other abnormality.
466. See the translation by Selby (2005, 265) of Ca.Śā.8.31.

467. *Pippalividaṅgaṭaṅkaṇasamacūrṇaṃ yā pibet payasā | ṛtusamaye na hi tasyā garbhaḥ sañjāyate kvāpi ||33||* *Piper Longum—pippalī*. See Sivarajan and Balachandran 1994, 374–376. *Embelia ribes—viḍaṅga*. See Sivarajan and Balachandran 1994, 507–510. Borax—*ṭaṅkaṇa*. See Nadkarni 1954, 103–108.
468. *Āranālaparipeṣitaṃ tryahaṃ yā japākusumam atti puṣpiṇī | satpurāṇaguḍamuṣṭisevinī sandadhāti na hi garbham aṅganā ||34||*. It should be noted that the eleven to fourteen days following the onset of menstruation was considered the time in which a woman could conceive. See Das (2003, 14f.) on a woman's period of fecundity according to ancient Indian medical literature.
469. See Meulenbeld 1999–2002, II A, 251.
470. See Meulenbeld 1999–2002, II A, 300–301.
471. See Meulenbeld 1999–2002, II A, 319.
472. See Meulenbeld 1999–2002, II A, 326.
473. See Meulenbeld 1999–2002, II A, 351. For a list of publications on ayurvedic contraceptives and abortifacient drugs, see Meulenbeld 1999–2002, II B, 374, note 514.
474. See Dossi, (1998, 121) for the Sanskrit text and German translation of the relevant verses.
475. See Young (1989).
476. On the modern debate about letting die and killing, physician-assisted suicide, and voluntary active euthanasia, see Beauchamp and Childress (2001, 139–152).
477. This follows the reasoning laid out in Ca.Sū.10.5, where Ātreya claims that a good physician will always be able to effect cure where cure is possible.
478. See, for example, chapters 4–6. in Ca.Si.
479. See Ca.Si.4.55 and Ca.Si.6.94.
480. Cakrapāṇidatta *ad* Ca.Sū.8.19 in reference to Ca.Cik.8.19.
481. See Bhāv.Pūrv.6.53.
482. Ca.Sū.9.26, Ca.Cik.1.58 and As.Utt.50.196.
483. Su.Sū.25.43–44.
484. As.Utt.50.189.
485. There is one exception: In Kaśyapa's description of a physician's professional conduct, he briefly notes that a physician should always comfort a patient. See Kāś.Vi.2(?).8.
486. Ca.Sū.15.11.
487. Su.Sū.10.4.
488. Ca.Cik.1.59. The same verse also occurs in As.Utt.50.190.
489. Ca.Sū.30.29.
490. Kāś.Vi.2(?).10, middle part.
491. See Manu. 1.87–91.

492. Ca.Cik.1.58, my own translation, and Ca.Cik.1.62, translation by Dominik Wujastyk (1993, 762).
493. See Wujastyk 2004b, 836. "Righteousness" here refers to the brahmanic concept of *dharma* in the sense of living according to the rules set out in the *Dharmaśāstras.*
494. Preisendanz notes that one of the findings of the Vienna project working on a critical edition of the *Carakasaṃhitā* is that "we could ascertain that in the core-group of mss. belonging to the Kashmir tradition, which seems to take us back to a rather old version of the text (compared with the majority of the other branches of the tradition that can be discerned) the well-known formula *iti ha smāha bhagavān ātreyaḥ* is not found at the beginning of the individual chapters within a *sthāna.*" (Diacritics and italics added. Email to Classical Ayurveda Working Group, July 18, 2007.)
495. In the edition by Srikantha Murthy (1998–), the *sa* is part of a compound with *cikitsya,* which I think is incorrect.
496. Cf. Śār.Pūrv.3.15, which is almost identical.
497. See Su.Sū.34.21cd–22ab.
498. Srikantha Murthy's edition of the *Bhāvaprakāśa* reads *bhiṣagvidhāḥ* instead of *bhiṣagvidā.* However, this verse is a quote from Ca.Si.2.4–6, which reads *bhiṣagvidā* according to Trikamji's edition.
499. See Sār.Pūrv.3.12.
500. See Su.Sū.34.19cd–21ab.
501. See Su.Sū.34.24.
502. See Su.Sū.34.22–23.
503. Note that Trikamjī reads *tīvrādharmārucer* instead of *tīvrādharmarucer* in the main text but gives the second reading in his rendering of Cakrapāṇidatta's commentary.
504. All of the above copies Ca.Sū.29.7 on the "savers of life."
505. "*Kalyāṇe kalyāṇe ca karaṇe maitre muhūrte*" is shortened to "*kalyāṇe muhūrte,*" "at an auspicious time," in the critical edition of the Vienna project. There are also many divergences in the following sentences, though these mostly consist of a change in the order of words and not so much in a change in the general meaning of the passage.
506. This sentence, beginning with *brahmacāriṇā,* is recorded as an interpolation in the Viennese critical edition.
507. Tewari makes note of the variant reading *saṃyatakeśa,* but uses *saṃhatakeśa* in her translation.
508. Tewari makes note of *praviśet* as a variant reading to *pradiśet* but uses the former in her translation.
509. The *Aṣṭāṅgasaṃgraha* has a parallel passage in Sūtrasthāna 3.38cd–40ab.

Bibliography

Achaya, K. T. (1998). *A Historical Dictionary of Indian Food.* New Delhi: Oxford University Press.

Ainslie, Whitelaw (1813). *Materia Medica of Hindoostan and Artisan's and Agriculturist's Nomenclature.* Madras: Government of Madras Press.

——— (1826). *Materia Indica: or Some Account of Those Articles Which Are Employed [by] the Hindoos and Other Eastern Nations in Their Medicine, Arts, and Agriculture.* London: Longman.

Arnold, David (1993). *Colonizing the Body: State Medicine and Epidemic Disease in Nineteenth-Century India.* Berkeley: University of California Press.

Athavale, V. B., and K. V. Athavale (2003). *The Ideal Physician.* Chaukhamba Ayurvijnan Studies 20. Delhi: Chaukhamba Sanskrit Pratishthan.

Banerjee, Madhulika (1995). "Power, Culture, Medicine: A Study of Ayurvedic Pharmaceuticals in India." Ph.D. diss., University of Delhi, Department of Political Science.

Basham, A. L. (1967). *The Wonder That Was India.* 3rd ed. London: Sidgwick & Jackson.

——— (1998 [1976]). "The Practice of Medicine in Ancient and Medieval India." In Leslie (1998 [1976]), 18–43.

Beauchamp, Tom L., and James F. Childress (2001). 5th ed. *Principles of Biomedical Ethics.* Oxford: Oxford University Press.

Benner, Dagmar (2005a). "Healing and Medicine in Ayurveda and South Asia." In Lindsay Jones (ed.), *Encyclopedia of Religion,* 3852–3858. 2nd ed. New York: MacMillan.

——— (2005b). "The Medical Ethics of Professionalized Ayurveda." *Asian Medicine: Tradition and Modernity* 1(1).

——— (2009). "*Saṃskāras* in Vāgbhaṭa's *Aṣṭāṅgahṛdayasaṃhitā*: *Garbhādhāna, ṛtusaṃgamana, puṃsavana.*" In Dominik Wujastyk (ed.), *Mathematics and Medicine in Sanskrit,* vol. 7 of *Papers of the 12th World Sanskrit Conference,* 119–138. Delhi: Motilal Banarsidass.

Bode, Maarten (2008). *Taking Traditional Knowledge to the Market: The Modern Image of the Ayurvedic and Unani Industry, 1980–2000.* New perspectives in South Asian history 21. Hyderabad: Orient Longman. Originally Ph.D. diss., University of Amsterdam, 2004.

Bodewitz, H. W. (2003). "The Concept of Sampad in the Arthaśāstra, the Vedic Prose Texts and the Gītā." *Indo-Iranian Journal,* 46(3): 231–259.

Chattopadhyaya, Debiprasad (1977). *Science and Society in Ancient India.* Calcutta: Research India Publication.

Cordier, Palmyr (1989). "L'enseignement médical dans L'Inde ancienne. Temps védico-brahmanique." In Arion Roşu (ed.), *Un demi-siècle de recherches āyurvédiques. Gustave Liétard et Palmyr Cordier: Travaux sur l'histoire de la médecine indienne,* 497–511. Paris: Institut de Civilisation Indienne.

Coward, Harold G., Julius J. Lipner, and Katherine K. Young (1989). *Hindu Ethics: Abortion, Purity and Euthanasia.* McGill studies in the history of religions, Albany: State University of New York Press.

Crawford, Cromwell (2003). *Hindu Bioethics for the Twenty-First Century.* New York: SUNY Press.

Das, Rahul Peter (2003). *The Origin of the Life of a Human Being: Conception and the Female According to Ancient Indian Medical and Sexological Literature.* Vol. 6 of *Indian Medical Tradition.* Delhi: Motilal Banarsidass.

Desai, Prakash N. (1989). *Health and Medicine in the Hindu Tradition: Continuity and Cohesion.* New York: Crossroad.

——— (1995). "Medical Ethics, History of: South and South East Asia. B. India." In Warren Thomas Reich (ed.), *Encyclopedia of Bioethics,* vols. 1–5, 1471–1476. 3rd ed. New York: Simon & Schuster Macmillan.

Deshpande, Madhav M. (1993). *Sanskrit & Prakrit: Sociolinguistic Issues,* vol. 6 of *MLBD Series in Linguistics.* Delhi: Motilal Banarsidass.

Dossi, Beatrice (1998). *Samen, Seele, Blut: Die Zeugungstheorien des alten Indiens.* Munich.

Filliozat, Jean (1964). *The Classical Doctrine of Indian Medicine.* New Delhi: Munshiram Manoharlal.

Francis, C. M. (1997). "Medical Ethics in India: Ancient and Modern (II)." *Issues in Medical Ethics* 5(1). Consulted at www.issuesinmedicalethics.org/051ed003html.

Gonda, Jan (1980). *Vedic Ritual: The Non-solemn Rites.* Leiden: Brill.

Griffiths, Mark (1994). *The New Horticultural Society Index of Garden Plants.* London: Macmillan.

Hessler, Franz (1844–55). *Ayurvédas: Id est medicinae systema a venerabili D'Hanvantare demonstratum a Susruta discipulo compositum; Nunc primum ex Sanskrita in Latinum sermonem vertit, introductionem, annotationes et rerum indice Franciscus Hessler.* Erlangen: Ferdinandum Enke.

Heyne, Benjamin (1814). *Tracts, historical and statistical, on India: With journals of several tours through various parts of the peninsula; also, an account of Sumatra, in a series of letters.* London: Printed for Robert Baldwin . . . , and Black, Parry, and Co. booksellers to the Hon. East India Company.

Hilgenberg, Luise, and Willibald Kirfel (1941). *Vāgbhaṭa's Aṣṭāṅgahṛdayasaṃhitā, ein altindisches Lehrbuch der Heilkunde, aus dem Sanskrit ins Deutsche übertragen mit Einleitung, Anmerkungen und Indices.* Leiden: Brill.

Hillebrandt, Alfred (1897). *Ritual-Litteratur. Vedische Opfer und Zauber,* vol. 3.2 of *Grundriss der indo-arischen Philologie und Altertumskunde.* Strassburg.

Hopkins, Edward Washburn (1932). "The Oath in Hindu Epic Literature." *Journal of the American Oriental Society* 52: 316–337.

Huguet, Gérard (1993). *La Medicine Indienne Traditionelle et la Fin de la Vie: Considerations Ethiques et Medicales. Interet Pratique Actuel.* Diplome d'etat de docteur en medicine, Université de Bordeaux II, Bordeaux.

Jaggi, O. P. (1982). "Medical Ethics, History of: India." In Warren Thomas Reich (ed.), *Encyclopedia of Bioethics,* vols. 1–4, 906–911. 2nd ed. New York: Free Press.

Jee, Bhagvat Sinh (1896). *A Short History of Aryan Medical Science.* London: Macmillan.

Jolly, Julius (1994 [1951]). *Indian Medicine, Translated from the German ... by C. G. Kashikar.* 3rd ed. New Delhi: Munshiram Manoharlal. First published 1951.

Jolly, Julius Ernst (1901). *Medicin.* Grundr. d. indo-ar. Philol. u. Altertumskunde Bd.3, Heft 10, Strassburg.

Jonsen, Albert R. (2000). *A Short History of Medical Ethics.* Oxford: Oxford University Press.

Kane, P. V. (1968–77). *A History of Dharmaśāstra.* 2nd ed. 5 vols. Poona: Bhandarkar Oriental Research Institute.

Kangle, R. P. (1972). *The Kauṭilīya Arthaśāstra.* 2nd ed. 3 vols. Delhi: Motilal Banarsidass.

Kautilya (1987). *The Arthashastra. Edited, Rearranged, Translated and Introduced by L. N. Rangarajan.* New Delhi: Penguin Books.

Krishnamurthy, K. H. (2000). *Bhela-Saṃhitā. Text with English Translation, Commentary and Critical notes.* No. 8 in Haridas Ayurveda Series, Varanasi: Chaukhambha Visvabharati.

Kuṃṭe, Aṇṇā Moreśvara, Kṛṣṇaśāstrī Navare, and Hariśāstrī Parādkar (eds.) (1995). *Aṣṭāṅgahṛdayam, śrīmadvāgbhaṭaviracitam, śrīmadaruṇadattaviracitayā "sarvāṅgasundaryākhyā" vyākhyayā hemādripraṇītayā "āyurvedarasāyanāhvayā" ṭīkayā ca samullasitam.* No. 4 in Kṛṣṇadāsa Āyurveda Sīrīja, Vārāṇasī: Krishnadas Academy. Reprint.

de La Vallée Poussin, Louis (1936–37). "Le Bouddhisme at le Yoga de Patañjali." *Mélanges chinois et bouddhiques* 28(5): 223–242.

Lal, Vinay (2005). *The History of History: Politics and Scholarship in Modern India.* Delhi: Oxford India Paperbacks.

Lavekar, G. S. (1996). *Doctor-Patient Relationship in Ancient Indian Medicine (Ayurveda).* Chaukhamba Sanskrit Bhawan Series No. 9. Varanasi: Chauwkhamba Sanskrit Bhawan.

Leslie, Charles (ed.) (1998 [1976]). *Asian Medical Systems: A Comparative Study.* Indian Medical Tradition 3. Delhi: Motilal Banarsidass.

Leslie, Julia, and Dominik Wujastyk (1991). "The Doctor's Assistant: Nursing in Ancient Indian Medical Texts." In Pat Holden and Jenny Littlewood (eds.), *Anthropology and Nursing*, 25–30. London: Routledge.

Liétard, Gustave (1858). "Essai sur l'histoire de la médicine chez les Indous." Ph.D. Diss. Reprinted in Roşu 1989, 5–62.

——— (1862). *Lettres historiques sur la médecine chez les Indous.* Paris: Victor Masson et Fils. Reprinted in Roşu 1989, 63–140.

——— (1864?). "Suşruta." In *Dictionnaire encyclopédique des sciences médicales publié sous la direction de A. Dechambre*, 634–675. Paris: P. Asselin, Sr. de Labé, V. Masson et Fils. Reprinted in Roşu 1989, 141–180.

Lipner, Julius J. (1989). "The Classical Hindu View on Abortion and the Moral Status of the Unborn." In Coward et al. (1989), chap. 2.

Maas, Philipp A. (2006). *Samādhipāda: Das erste Kapitel des Pātañjalayogaśāstra zum ersten Mal kritisch ediert.* Vol. 9 of *Geisteskultur Indiens: Texte und Studien; Indologica Halensis.* Aachen: Shaker. Dissertation Bonn, Univ., 2004.

——— (2009). "The Concepts of the Human Body and Disease in Classical Yoga and Āyurveda." *Wiener Zeitschrift für die Kunde Südasiens* 51: 123–162.

Magner, Lois N. (1997). *Doctors, Nurses, and Medical Practitioners: A Bio-bibliographical Sourcebook.* Westport, Conn. Greenwood Press. Includes bibliographic references and index.

Maithrimurthi, Mudagamuwe (1999). *Wohlwollen, Mitleid, Freude und Gleichmut: Eine ideengeschichtliche Untersuchung der vier apramāṇas in der buddhistischen Ethik und Spiritualität von den Anfangen bis hin zum frühen Yogācāra.* Vol. 50 of Alt- und neu-indische Studien. Stuttgart: Steiner.

Malamoud, Charles (2002). "Doctors as Characters in Sanskrit Narrative Literature." In Ana Salema (ed.), *Āyurveda at the Crossroads of Care and Cure: Proceedings of the Indo-European Seminar on Ayurveda held at Arrábida, Portugal, in November 2001*, 24–30. Lisbon: Centro de História del Além-Mar, Universidade Nova de Lisboa.

Mazars, Guy (1995). *La médecine indienne.* Que Sais-je? Paris: Presses Universitaires de France.

——— (2006). *A Concise Introduction to Indian Medicine.* Vol. 8 of *Indian Medical Tradition.* Delhi: Motilal Banarsidass.

Menon, I. A., and H. F. Haberman (1970). "The Medical Students' Oath of Ancient India." *Medical History* 14: 295–299.

Meulenbeld, Gerrit Jan (1974). *The Mādhavanidāna and Its Chief Commentary: Chapters 1–10. Introduction, Translation, and Notes.* Leiden: Brill.

——— (1987). "Reflections on the Basic Concepts of Indian Pharmacology." In Gerrit Jan Meulenbeld and Dominik Wujastyk (eds.), *Studies on Indian Medical History*, 1–17. Groningen: Forsten.

——— (1999–2002). *A History of Indian Medical Literature.* 5 vols. Groningen: E. Forsten.

——— (2008). *The Mādhavanidāna with "Madhukośa," the Commentary by Vijayarakṣita and Śrīkaṇṭhadatta (Ch. 1–10). Introduction, Translation, and Notes.* 2nd ed. Indian Medical Tradition, New Delhi: Motilal Banarsidass.

Monier-Williams, Monier (1993). A Sanskrit – English Dictionary Etymologically and Philologically Arranged with Special Reference to Caognate Indo–European Languages. New Edition, Geatly Enlarged and Improved. Delhi: Motical Banarsidass Publish Private Limited.

Mookerji, Radha Kumud (1947). *Ancient Indian Education (Brahmanical and Buddhist).* London: Macmillan.

Müller, R. F. G. (1934). "On Sattva, Rajas and Tamas in the Old Indian Medicine." *Journal of Ayurveda* 10(8): 295–302.

Nadkarni, A. K. (1954). *Dr. K. M. Nadkarni's Indian Materia Medica, with Ayurvedic, Unani-tibbi, Siddha, Allopathic, Homeopathic, Naturopathic & Home Remedies, Appendices & Notes.* 2 vols. Bombay: Popular Prakashan.

Norman, K. R. (1992). *The Group of Discourses (Sutta-Nipāta). Vol. 2. Revised Translation with Introduction and Notes.* Pali Text Society Translation Series No. 45, Oxford: Pali Text Society.

Nutton, Vivian (2004). *Ancient Medicine.* Series of Antiquity. London: Routledge.

Oberlies, Thomas (2002). "Milch und Soma: Die Formalien eines Vertragsschlusses." *Studien zur Indologie und Iranistik* 23: 71–90.

Oldenberg, Hermann (1886). *The Grihya-Sūtras. Rules of Vedic Domestic Ceremonies.* Pt. 1, *Sankhayana-Grihya-Sutra; Asvalayana-Grihya-Sutra; Paraskara-Grihya-Sutra; Khadira-Grihya-Sutra.* No. 29 in Sacred Books of the East, Oxford: Clarendon Press.

Olivelle, Patrick (1999). *Dharmasūtras. The Law Codes of Ancient India. A New Translation by Patrick Olivelle.* World's Classics. Oxford: Oxford University Press.

——— (2005). *Manu's Code of Law. A Critical Edition and Translation of the Mānava-Dharmaśāstra.* South Asia Research. Oxford: Oxford University Press.

Pandya, S. K. (1999). "Medical Ethics in India: Then and Now." In H. August van Alphen, (ed.), *Neurosurgery and Medical Ethics*, 35–46. New York: Springer.

Pollock, Sheldon (1985). "The Theory of Practice and the Practice of Theory in Indian Intellectual History." *Journal of the American Oriental Society* 3(105): 499–519.

——— (1989). "Mīmāṃsā and the Problem of History in Traditional India." *Journal of the American Oriental Society* 109(4): 603–610.

Preisendanz, Karin (2007). "The Initiation of the Medical Student in Early Classical Āyurveda: Caraka's Treatment in Context." In Karin Preisendanz (ed.), *Expanding and Merging Horizons: Contributions to South Asian and Cross-cultural Studies in Commemoration of Wilhelm Halbfass.* Vienna: Verlag der Oesterreichischen Akademie der Wissenschaften.

——— (2009). "Logic, Debate and Epistemology in Ancient Indian Medicine and Philosophy—an Investigation." *Indian Journal of History of Science* 44(2): 261–312.

Prets, Ernst, and Joachim Prandstetter (1991–). *Terminologie der frühen philosophischen Scholastik in Indien: Ein Begriffswörterbuch zur altindischen Dialektik, Erkenntnislehre und Methodologie.* Österreichische Akademie der Wissenschaften, Philosophisch-Historische Klasse, Denkschriften, 223, band 1–2. Vienna: Verlag der Österreicheischen Akademie der Wissenschaften. Band 1 (1991): A–I, Band 2 (1996): U–Pū.

Puschmann, Theodor (ed.) (1891). *A History of Medical Education from the Most Remote to the Most Recent Times.* London: H. K. Lewis.

Raghavan, V., K. Kunjunni Raja, C. S. Sundaram, N. Veezhinathan, and N. Gangadharan (1949–). *New Catalogus Catalogorum, an Alphabetical Register of Sanskrit and Allied Works and Authors.* Madras University Sanskrit Series, Madras: University of Madras. References to vol.1 are to the revised 1968 edition.

Raison, Alix (1974). *La Hāritasaṃhitā: Texte médical sanskrit.* Publications de l'Institut français d'indologie; no. 52. Pondicherry: Institut français d'indologie.

Ramachandra Rao, S. K., and S. R. Sudarshan (1985–87). *Encylopaedia of Indian Medicine.* Bombay: Popular Prakashan.

Roşu, Arion (1989). *Un demi-siècle de recherches āyurvédiques. Gustave Liétard et Palmyr Cordier: Travaux sur l'histoire de la médecine indienne.* Paris: Institut de Civilisation Indienne.

Roth, Rudolph (1872). "Indische Medicin. Caraka." *Zeitschrift der Deutschen Morgenländischen Gesellschaft* 26: 441–452.

Scharfe, Hartmut (1999). "The Doctrine of the Three Humors in Traditional Indian Medicine and the Alleged Antiquity of Tamil Siddha Medicine." *Journal of the American Oriental Society* 119(4): 609–629.

——— (2002). *Education in Ancient India.* No. 2: South Asia, 16 in Handbuch der Orientalistik. Leiden: Brill.

Selby, Martha Ann (2005). "Narratives of Conception, Gestation, and Labour in Sanskrit Āyurvedic Texts." *Asian Medicine, Tradition and Modernity,* 1(2): 254–275.

Sharma, Priya Vrat (1999–2001). *Suśruta-Saṃhitā, with English Translation of Text and Ḍalhaṇa's Commentary Alongwith [sic] Critical Notes.* 3 vols. Vol. 9 of *Haridas Ayurveda Series.* Varanasi: Chaukhambha Visvabharati.

——— (2003). *Caraka-Saṃhitā: Agniveśa's Treatise Refined and Annotated by Caraka and Redacted by Dṛḍhabala (Text with English Translation).* 4 vols. Delhi: Chaukhambha Orientalia.

Siegel, Lee (1985). "How Many Vaidyas Does It Take to Change a Lightbulb? The Satire of Physicians in Sanskrit Literature." *Bulletin d'Études Indiennes* 3: 167–193.

——— (1987). *Laughing Matters: Comic Tradition in India.* Chicago: University of Chicago Press.

Singhal, G. D., and Pt. Damodar Sharma Gaur (1963). *Surgical Ethics in Āyurveda.* Chowkhamba Sanskrit Studies. Vol. 40. Varanasi: Vidya Vilas Press.

Sivarajan, V. V., and Indira Balachandran (1994). *Ayurvedic Drugs and Their Plant Sources.* New Delhi: Oxford & IBH.

Smith, Frederick M. (2006). *The Self-Possessed: Deity and Spirit Possession in South Asian Literature and Civilization.* New York: Columbia University Press.

Srikantha Murthy, K. R. (1991–95). *Vāgbhaṭa's Aṣṭāṅga Hṛdayam: Text, English Translation, Notes, Appendix, and Indices.* 3 vols. Varanasi: Krishnadas Academy.

——— (1993). *Mādhava Nidānam (Roga Viniscaya) of Madhavakara (a Treatise on Āyurveda). Text with English Translation, Critical Introduction and Appendices.* Delhi: Chaukhambha Orientalia.

——— (1995–97). *Aṣṭāṅga Samgraha of Vāgbhaṭa: Text, English Translation, Notes, Indices etc.* 3 vols. Varanasi: Chaukhambha Orientalia.

——— (1998–). *Bhāvaprakāśa of Bhāvamiśra (Text, English Translation, Notes, Appendices, and Index).* Varanasi: Krishnadas Academy. One volume published to date.

Staal, Frits (2008). *Discovering the Vedas.* New Delhi: Penguin Books India.

Subrahmanya Ayyar, K. V. (1984). "The Tirumukkudal Inscription of Virarajendra." In *Epigraphia Indica,* vol. 21, 1931–32, chap. 38, 220–250. Calcutta: Superintendent of Government Printing. Reprinted 1984.

Tewari, Premvati (1996). *Kāśyapa-saṃhitā or Vṛddhajīvakīya Tantra: Text with English Translation and Commentary.* Varanasi: Chaukhambha Visvabharati.

Trautmann, Thomas R. (1971). *Kauṭilya and the Arthaśāstra: A Statistical Investigation of the Authorship and Evolution of the Text.* Leiden: Brill.

Trikamji Ācārya, Jādavji (ed.) (1992a). *Carakasaṃhitā, śrīcakrapāṇidattaviracitayā āyurvedadīpikāvyākhyayā saṃvalitā.* 5th ed. New Delhi: Munshiram Manoharlal.

——— (1992b). *Suśrutasaṃhitā, śrīḍalhaṇācāryaviracitayā nibandhasaṃgrahākhyavyākhyayā nidānasthānasya śrīgayadāsācāryaviracitayā nyāyacandrikākhyapañjikāvyākhyayā ca samullasitā ... Ācāryopāhvena trivikramātmajena yādavaśarmaṇā ... saṃśodhitā.* 5th ed. Delhi: Caukhambhā Oriyanṭāliyā.

Valiathan, M. S. (2007). *The Legacy of Suśruta.* Chennai: Orient Longman.

——— (2003). *The Legacy of Caraka.* Chennai: Orient Longman.

Vidyasagar, Parashuram Shastri (1986). *The Śārṅgadhara-Saṃhitā by Paṇḍita Śārṅgadharāchārya Son of Paṇḍita Damodara with the commentaries. Adhamalla's "Dipika" and Kashirama's "Gudhartha-Dipika."* Edited with footnotes. Krishnadas Ayurveda Series 14. Varanasi: Krishnadas Academy.

Warrier, P. K., V. P. K. Nambiar, and C. Ramankutty (eds.) (1994–96). *Indian Medicinal Plants: A Compendium of 500 Species. Vaidyaratnam P. S. Varier's Arya Vaidya Sala, Kottakal.* 5 vols. Madras: Orient Longman.

Wezler, A. (2003). "Sampad of Bhagavadgītā XVI Reconsidered." In *Harānandalaharī: Volume in Honour of Professor Minoru Hara on His Seventieth Birthday,* 433–455. Reinbek: Dr. Inge Wezler Verlag für Orientalistische Fachpublikationen.

Wezler, Albrecht (1984). "On the Quadruple Division of the Yogaśāstra, the Caturvyūhatva of the Cikitsāśāstra and the 'Four Noble Truths' of the Buddha." *Indologica Taurinensia* 12: 289–337.

Wilson, H. H. (1823). "Medical and Surgical Sciences of the Hindus." *Asiatic Journal and Monthly Register for British India and Its Dependencies* 16: 207–212, 349–356.

Wise, Thomas A. (1845). *Commentary on the Hindu System of Medicine.* Calcutta: Thacker.

Woodward, F. L., E. M. Hare, and Pali Text Society (1986–92). *The Book of the Gradual Sayings: Anguttara-Nikāya, or, More-Numbered Suttas.* Translation series no. 22, 24–27. Reprint. London: Pali Text Society. Originally published: London: Luzac, 1932–36.

Wujastyk, Dominik (1993). "Indian Medicine." In W. F. Bynum and Roy Porter (eds.), *Companion Encyclopedia of the History of Medicine,* vol. 1, chap. 33, 755–778. 2 vols. London: Routledge.

——— (2003). *The Roots of Āyurveda: Selections from Sanskrit Medical Writings.* 3rd updated ed., London Penguin Group.

——— (2004a). "Agni and Soma: A Universal Classification." *Studia Asiatica: International Journal for Asian Studies* 4–5: 347–370.

——— (2004b). "Medicine and Dharma." *Journal of Indian Philosophy* 32(5): 831–842.

——— (2007–8). "Post-classical Indian Traditions of Medical Debate and Argumentation." *eJournal of Indian Medicine* 2(3): 67–81.

——— (in preparation). "The *Rogārogavāda* of Vīreśvara: A Critical Edition and Translation."

Young, Katherine K. (1989). "Euthanasia: Traditional Hindu Views and the Contemporary Debate." In Coward et al. (1989), chap. 3.

Zimmer, Henry R. (1948). *Hindu Medicine.* Baltimore: Johns Hopkins University Press. Posthumous publication.

Zimmermann, Francis (1999 [1987]). *The Jungle and the Aroma of Meats: An Ecological Theme in Hindu Medicine.* Vol. 4 of *Indian Medical Tradition.* Delhi: Motilal Banarsidass. Originally published Berkeley: University of California Press, 1987.

Zysk, Kenneth G. (1998 [1991]). *Asceticism and Healing in Ancient India: Medicine in the Buddhist Monastery,* vol. 2 of *Indian Medical Tradition.* 2nd ed. Delhi: Motilal Banarsidass. Originally published 1991.

——— (1999). "Mythology and the Brāhmaṇization of Indian Medicine: Transforming Heterodoxy into Orthodoxy." In Folke Josephson (ed.), *Categorisation and Interpretation,* 125–145. Göteborg: Meijerbergs institut för svensk etymologisk forskning, Göteborgs universitet.

——— (2000). *Asceticism and Healing in Ancient India: Medicine in the Buddhist Monastery.* Vol. 2 of *Indian Medical Tradition.* 3rd ed. Delhi: Motilal Banarsidass. Originally published 1991.

Index

www.ingramcontent.com/pod-product-compliance
Ingram Content Group UK Ltd.
Pitfield, Milton Keynes, MK11 3LW, UK
UKHW020923170926
475595UK00031B/47